TAI CHI CHUAN

Roots and Branches

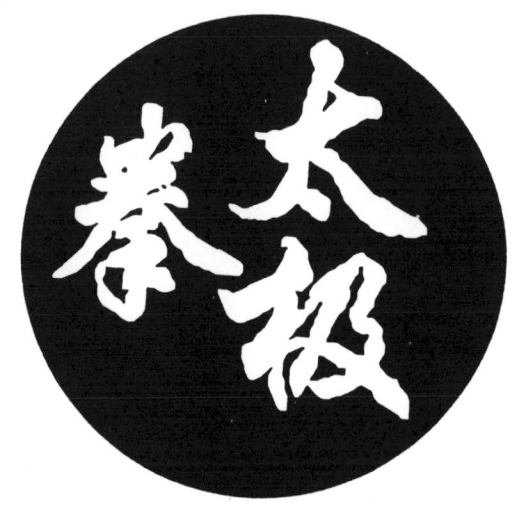

Nigel Sutton

CHARLES E. TUTTLE COMPANY
Rutland, Vermont & Tokyo, Japan

Heartfelt thanks are due to all my teachers and students without whom this book would not have been possible. A special thank you also to Mr. Teng Beng Kit for his beautiful artwork.

Published by the Charles E. Tuttle Company, Inc.
of Rutland, Vermont & Tokyo, Japan
with editorial offices at
2-6 Suido 1-chome, Bunkyo-ku, Tokyo 112

First edition published 1993
by Perfect Balance Books, Johor, Malaysia

LCC Card No. 96-60595
ISBN 0-8048-2072-4

First Tuttle edition, 1996
Reprinted, 1997

Printed in Singapore

This book is greatfully dedicated to
Master Liang He Ching
who taught me what it means to be a teacher
and to Master Koh Ah Tee

" Things have their root and their branches.
Affairs have their end and their beginning.
To know what is first and what is last
will lead near to what is taught."
Confucius.

Wherever "he" or "him" are used in the text, this should
be understood to also stand for "she" or "her."

Table of Contents

Introduction   1

Roots   2

Part One: Form
Chishi—Beginning   8
Zuo Peng—Left Ward Off   11
You Lan Jue Wei (Peng, Lu, Ji, An)—Grasp the Sparrow's Tail (Ward
   Off, Rollback, Press, and Push)   13
Zhuan Shen Diao Shou—Turn Body and Drop the Hands   21
Dan Bian—Single Whip   23
Ti Shou Shang Shi—Lift Hands   25
Kao—Shoulder strike   27
Bai He Liang Chi—White Crane Spread Its Wings   29
Lou Chi Ao Bu—Brush Knee Twist Step   31
Shou Hui Pipa—Strum the Lute   33
Lou Xi Ao Bu   35
Jing Bu Ban Lan Chui—Step Forward, Move, Parry, Punch   36
Rufeng Sibi—As if Closing a Door   38
Shizi Shou—Cross Hands   40
Bao Hu Gui Shan—Embrace Tiger, Return to Mountain   42
Xie Dan Bian—Diagonal Single Whip   44
Zhou Di Kan Chui—Fist Under Elbow   45
Dao Nian Hou—Step Back Repulse Monkey   48
Xie Fei Shi—Diagonal Flying   52
Yun Shou—Cloud Hands   54
Dan Bian Xia She—Single Whip, Low Form   56
Jing Ji Du Li—Golden Rooster Stands on One Leg   58
Zuo You Fen Jiao—Left and Right Toe Kick   60
Zhuan Shen Deng Jiao—Turn Body Heel Kick   63
Jing Bu Zai Chui—Step Forward and Plant a Punch   66
Jing Bu Lan Jue Wei—Step Forward Grasp the Sparrow's Tail   67

Dan Bian—Single Whip 68
Yu Nu Chuan Suo—Fair Lady Plays Shuttles 69
You Lan Jue Wei—Right Grasp the Sparrow's Tail 72
Shang Bu Qi Xing—Step Up to Seven Stars 74
Tui Bu Kua Hu—Step Back to Ride the Tiger 75
Zhuan Shen Bai Lian Tui—Turn Body White Lotus Kick 77
Wang Gong She Hu—Draw a Bow to Shoot the Tiger 79
Jing Bu Ban Lan Chui—Step Forward, Move, Parry, and Punch 80

Part Two: Branches

From Form to Function 82
Starting Points: Applying the Form 84
Chi Shi—Beginning 84
Peng, Ti Shou Shang Shi, Yu Nu Chuan Suo—Ward-Off, Lift Hands, Fair Lady Grasps Shuttles 86
Jing Bu Ban Lan Chui—Step Forward, Move, Parry, Punch 88
Lu, Shou Hui Pipa—Rollback, Strum the Lute 90
Xie Fei Shi, Dan Bian—Diagonal Flying, Single Whip 92
Lou Xi Ao Bu—Brush Knee Twist Step 93
Tai Chi Kicking Technique 94
Yun Shou—Cloud hands 96
Bai He Liang Chi—White Crane Spreads Its Wings 96
Bao Hu Gui Shan—Embrace Tiger Return to Mountain 97
Jing Bu Zai Chui—Step Forward and Plant a Punch 98
Dao Nian Hou—Step Back Repulse Monkey 98
Zhou Di Kan Chui—Fist Under Elbow 99
Shang Bu Chi Xing, Tui Bu Gua Hu—Step Up to Seven Stars, Step Back to Ride a Tiger 100
Rufeng Sibi—Apparent Close Up 100
Shi Zi Shou—Cross Hands 101
Ji—Press 101
An—Push 101

Part Three: Gaining from the Experience of the Past

The Classics 102

Part Four: Signposts for the Path

Ng Kiong Hin 114
Tan Ching Ngee 116
Lau Kim Hong 118
Koh Ah Tee 120

TAI CHI CHUAN
ROOTS AND BRANCHES

Introduction

This book contains detailed instruction on how to perform what is probably the most widely practised tai chi routine in the world, that developed by Master Cheng Man Ching. But it is not just a book about physical movement for it gives the practitioner a wealth of information concerning both the whys and wherefores of the art and practical exercises that may be performed both solo and with a partner, with the ultimate aim of enriching the tai chi experience of both novice and advanced practitioner.

Although the solo form is both the starting point and the destination, on the course of your journey through this book you will be introduced to many aspects of tai chi, and hopefully, on the way you will find much to stimulate your interest and to keep your study of the art fresh and rewarding.

In order to preserve that precious thread between the past and the present, a selection of advice from the "classic" teachings of the art is included, together with a commentary illustrating precisely how such teachings can be brought to life through practice of the form.

As you start your study of this book you will be embarking on a path already trod by tens of thousands of travellers and hopefully, like them you will enjoy every step of the way !

ROOTS

The solo form presented in this book is that developed by Professor Cheng Man Ching (1901-1975), who learnt from the renowned Yang family, and used his knowledge of Chinese art, medicine and philosophy to create his own thirty-seven posture form. The fact that this form is considerably shorter than the traditional Yang style form, which is comprised of 108 postures, offers its practitioners a number of advantages.

The first of these lies in its very shortness, as we can run through the whole form without losing sight of our particular training objective. All of us, as human beings, have limited attention spans. Even at the slowest pace the Cheng Man Ching form should only take about twelve minutes, which most of us can cope with. Let us imagine, for example, that we want to practise the form, paying specific attention to allowing every movement to be directed by the waist; as the form is short enough to allow us to retain this thought as we practise, we can apply this principle to the whole form. Indeed when I used to practise the traditional form I would often find that I had got two-thirds of the way through the form, and had forgotten what exactly I was trying to practise! Thus I seldom applied the very principles that I wanted to practise to the whole form.

The second advantage of the thirty-seven posture form lies in the way it was developed to encapsulate all the important facets of the traditional form, while at the same time placing a great emphasis on the fundamental principle of relaxation. Professor Cheng eliminated what he felt to be the unnecessary repetitions in the form, contending that there was no point in them (see chapter V "Cheng Man Ching's Advanced Form Instructions" compiled and translated by Douglas Wile, Published by Sweet Ch'i Press 1985). There is not a single movement principle to be found embodied in any posture from the traditional form that does not appear in the thirty-seven posture form.

Bearing in mind that the whole routine is based on the need to develop the unique relaxation required of the tai chi chuan practitioner, let us go on examine how form practise is to be approached, in more detail.

When you start your practise of the form you must always bear in mind the importance of the principles it embodies rather than the applications that it illustrates. Furthermore each time that you do the form you should be aiming for perfection. It is as if you are painting a picture on a clean, new, fresh piece of paper. But before you actually start you must ensure that you are properly prepared.

The first part of this preparation is mental and consists of quieting your mind, expanding your consciousness to encompass the whole body and the environment that you are practising in, while at the same time still focussing on specific details. This mindset is absolutely vital if you are to make the art work for you.

The first step towards achieving the requisite state of mind consists of running through a mental checklist. I find it easiest to work systematically from the head downwards:

1) The head feels as if suspended from above
2) The eyes relax and look naturally forward but the student is also able to use his peripheral vision
3) The facial muscles relax
4) The mouth is held in a relaxed manner, or as the classic teachings state "not open, not closed"
5) The tip of the tongue is placed on the roof of the mouth
6) The shoulders are relaxed and naturally rounded
7) The back is naturally rounded and the chest naturally hollowed
8) There is an awareness of a slight space under the armpits
9) The elbow joints are relaxed and rounded
10) The fingers are open, "not straight and not bent"
11) The **tiger's mouth,** the area between the thumb and the index finger, feels slightly stretched

12) The waist feels relaxed and supple.
13) The backside is tucked under, so that the spine "hangs" naturally.
14) The knees are kept slightly bent.
15) The whole of the sole of the foot feels firmly connected to the floor.
16) The weight falls naturally through the front part of the foot, corresponding to the **yong quan** point in acupuncture.

Having run through this checklist you should do your best to feel as relaxed as possible, but always remembering that there is a structure underlying this relaxation. At this point, as you stand in a position of loose attention, prior to actually commencing the form, you might like to run through some of the key pieces of advice given in the "classics". Points to ponder might include:

1) Making the body like a needle concealed in cotton
2) Moving like a cat stalking its prey, gazing like an eagle
3) When one part moves the whole body moves
4) The flow of power is like silk reeling from a cocoon
5) The mind is placed in the **dantian** (an acupuncture point below the navel, corresponding to the body's centre of gravity)

While there are many other pieces of advice, the last one is a good point of departure as you start to move through the form.

Before you start it is worth reminding yourself of the reasons why the form is practised slowly. First of all you are moving at the pace which best allows you to check that each and every movement is correct. At the same time you are trying to "relax" into each posture. The slowness of movement also performs the vital function of allowing the mind to be in a state of "relaxed awareness". This mental state consists of the mind being able to concentrate on not concentrating ! If this sounds like so much nonsense it is because the practice of tai chi chuan is primarily about physical experience, and not the process of conceptualisation and verbalisation which must precede writing about the art.

One problem associated with the speed you practise the form arises from confusion over the "flowing" nature of the movements. Having trained extensively in the Far East it has become apparent to me that one major difference between the way Chinese students are taught to approach the art, and western students approach it, is in the matter of "flow". If you were to ask most non-Chinese their initial impression of tai chi chuan, it is usually of the flowing nature of the movements. Yet in the Far East the form is mostly taught "by the numbers", with students moving in almost mechanical fashion from one posture; or even from one part of a posture, to another. It is only the very advanced students who exhibit the "flow" which is allowed to develop in a very natural fashion and is not something particularly to be aimed for.

By way of contrast, almost from day one of their study, western students attempt to glide their way through the movements, which often results in many important points being missed. For example, it is very hard to actually learn about the finer points of balance when constantly moving through the "points" where the features of perfect balance can be illustrated and emphasised.

For the reasons described above it becomes obvious that exactly how slowly you practise the form depends upon your applying the factors above to your own training. Professor Cheng Man Ching was well known for the speed at which he ran through the form, but his recommendation was that it should take between seven and twelve minutes.

Once you have actually started the form your mind is busily involved in checking each posture, as well as generally checking the whole body for the appropriate measure of relaxation. This relaxation is the key thing, and you must constantly check every joint and every muscle to ensure that they are comfortable. This checking is guided by the advice that from the waist down should be full, while the upper body should remain light, empty and comfortable . This state of full and empty, however, is comparative, for in accordance with **yin-yang** philosophy, each individual arm and leg is alternately full and empty.

In order to check whether your posture is truly relaxed you are taught to hold a posture in a way which you are aware is not completely relaxed, and to take a deep breath. After which you should relax, as far as possible, into what you believe to be the correct stance, and again take a deep breath. Provided you have taken care to adjust your posture so as to maximise your ability to relax, you will find that the second breath not only feels more comfortable, but that it also feels as if the breath is deeper and lower down. In fact the feeling should be that you are actually breathing from the dantian, although, of course, physiologically speaking this is impossible.

The reason for this feeling of greater comfort is that by practising a relaxed posture that obeys the principles of the art, you will automatically ease any pressure that there might otherwise be on the ribcage, and this will allow the lungs to be used to their full capacity.

If you find that you frequently get out of breath when doing the form very often the cause is the positioning of the arms. If they are held too high the shoulders become tense and the ribcage becomes contracted thus restricting the natural action of the lungs.

You will find that as you progress in your study of the art your priorities in practising the form change according to the stage of development that you have reached. This progress tends to be cyclical rather than linear in nature. What this means is that in the early stages of your tai chi chuan career you might find that when you are practising you pay careful attention to the process of "rooting" (ensuring a firm connection to the ground); at a later stage you might find yourself returning to this same process as you realise there are deficiencies in your skill in this area.

What is it then that prompts the student to return again and again to their solo practice of the form? The answer lies in the way that the curriculum of the art is structured. As tai chi chuan teachers are often heard to say, the solo form teaches you to know yourself while pushing hands teaches you to know others. When the student learns pushing hands the weaknesses inherent in his form practice will be highlighted and graphically exemplified as he flies through the air !

At first you might find that there is a problem with your root, to return to the original example, so you will emphasise this when practising. When you have corrected this and your pushing hands skill has improved you might find that in placing emphasis on, for example, the use of your hands, your root has once again become faulty; and so, once again, when practising the form you have to emphasise rooting. This process of constant searching for ways to improve is a lifelong one, and one that ensures continual interest for there is always a new challenge to be faced and met!

As I have mentioned before the Cheng Man Ching form is not about specific self-defence applications, although it is important that you know what the movements are for, and how they might be used. What is far more important when you are practising, however, is the general principles embodied in these movements and we will now take a look at exactly what these principles are and what some of their purposes might be, as we work through the form.

PART 1 - FORM

Chishi - Beginning

When standing at the beginning it is best to use this opportunity to run through the checklist described earlier to ensure that your body is as relaxed as possible.

The first six leg and arm movements serve to direct your attention to the vital joints and the importance of relaxing and opening them. They are: the hip, knee and ankle in the leg and the shoulder, elbow and wrist in the arm. As you run though these moves all the joints in turn are opened and relaxed. At the same time your body sinks, the waist relaxes and you prepare yourself for the movements to follow.

As you stand quietly you should also relax your mind, endeavouring to focus completely on your movements. The first step in this mental preparation consists of "sinking the qi to the dantian". All that this piece of tai chi jargon means is that you should be aware of the dantian area, for according to Chinese thought where the mind goes the qi follows. What this serves to do in practical terms is to focus your attention on the centre of gravity This gives you a kind of mental anchor as you prepare to run though the form, and with time you will find that you develop the ability to remain mentally calm while thinking of several different things in close succession. This mental state is of vital importance if you are to use tai chi chuan as a martial art, for you must be prepared to respond to an opponent's attack while preserving your own state of calm.

Once you have achieved the appropriate mental state you may carry out the following moves:

You start the form standing in a loose attention position, hands by your sides, palms facing in and with your feet together, heels touching. Now is the time to run through your mental checklist, starting from the top of the head and working down.

First we carry out the six leg movements and then the six arm movements.

Transfer your weight to the right foot and then sink down by bending your right knee. As you drop allow the knee to sink down and in, naturally pivoting the left foot inwards on the toes. This ensures that your right hip and buttock remain relaxed. As you sink your palms turn to face the rear, fingers extended in the "fair lady's hand".

In the second move you turn your waist about forty-five degrees to the left allowing the legs to open as the left foot pivots out on the toe. This enables the left hip to remain loose and relaxed.

Next you step out with the left foot, placing it down heel first, a shoulder-width's distance away from the right foot. Then turn the foot to face forward, pivoting on the heel. Throughout this move the weight remains on the right foot.

Now you can simply shift the weight across to the left. This is the fourth move in the sequence.

The fifth move simply consists of turning the right foot, with the heel as the pivotal point, so that it faces directly forward.

The sixth and final move involving the legs is a simple shift of the weight to the right until it is distributed equally between them.

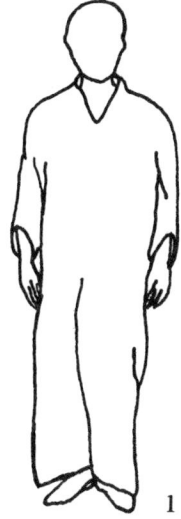

1

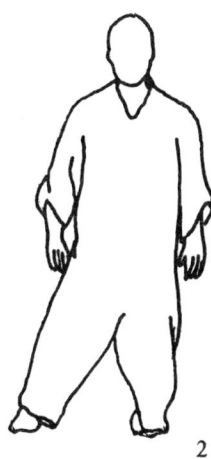

2

Next are the arm movements. Remember to keep your hands in the requisite position.

The first move is to raise both arms directly in front of you until the wrists are just above waist level, palms facing down. At this point you should feel as if your shoulder muscles are just about to start working. This we want to avoid at all times when doing tai chi.

To avoid this, sink both elbows. This is the second move.

From there raise the wrists up as if they were attached to wires until your hands are at approximately chest height.

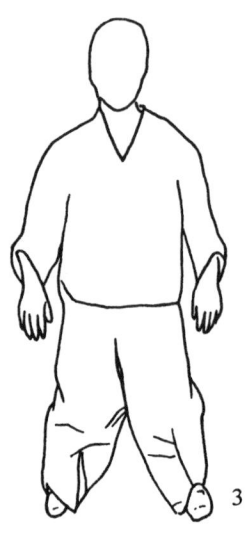

Next push your arms forward so that your fingers are rising up on a diagonal away from you. Again avoid engaging the shoulder muscles so stop when your wrists are at shoulder height.

The fifth move is to allow the arms to drop down at the sides to waist level, palms facing backwards and fingers facing down.

The final move consists of pushing down with the palms and then allowing the fingers to sink down so that your hands end up in the same position that they started from.

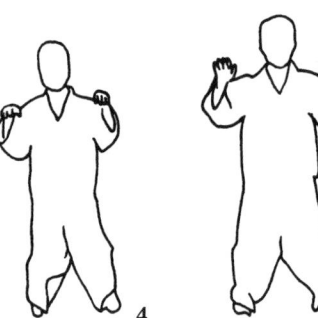

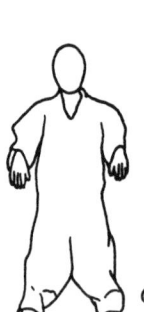

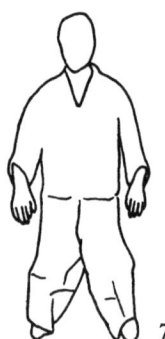

ZUO PENG - Left Ward Off

To move into this posture your waist turns to the right and your weight shifts on to the right leg. This begins the practice of shifting the weight on to one leg, "screwing" it into the ground, and in the process storing up the tai chi spring power of the legs and then releasing it into the next move. This is what Cheng Man Ching referred to as "swing and movement", whereby potential energy stored up from one movement is converted into kinetic energy producing the next movement. As in all the movements of the form the hands follow the turning of the waist.

As you move into the Left Ward-Off, the form teaches you to use the angles your body is creating. So, although the general "feel" of the movements is rounded, you are always seeking the straight line in the curve. In practical terms this can be seen in the transformations that occur as you move into left peng.

First the weight is on the right leg and the waist is turned to the right. Then the left leg steps out straight with the left hand following it forward. Next the waist is turned, bringing with it the back foot, pivoting on the heel, and turning the left hand so that the left forearm ends up facing front. So it is that within this one apparently simple movement occur a number of changes from curved to straight and back again. The whole movement is accomplished, however, with the bulk of the work being done by the legs and the waist. This feeling should be reproduced throughout your tai chi practice, so that the legs provide a platform for the free-moving, relaxed upper body. Bearing all this in mind you are now ready to perform ZUO PENG.

Having completed CHI SHI, shift your weight to the left leg, taking care that your hips remain on the same level. Then turn your waist to the right, allowing your right foot to pivot around on the heel through ninety degrees. At the same time your left hand moves around, following the waist at waist height, palm up, while the right arm raises up to chest height, palm down. Thus the two hands are placed as if holding a football in to the body. Take care that you keep the arms away from the body by making a space under both armpits. Now shift your weight to the right foot.

The left leg which remains firmly on the floor will now start to feel strained so allow the heel to raise and the knee to sink. Next you step out with the left leg directly to its front. You must make sure that you have stepped out far enough so that you will be able to form a front stance when the move is completed. About one and a half shoulder-widths is enough. As you step, the heel is put down first. Then shift your weight to the left leg, at the same time allowing the left hand and arm to rise up while the right arm drops at your side. The left arm moves up and out, with the palm facing in at about chest-height and the forearm about a shoulder width away from your chest. As in all the tai chi movements the elbows hang down.

Next you turn your waist to the left, to end up facing the same way as your stance. This waist movement causes the back foot to pivot on the heel to an angle of forty-five degrees. This will bring the left hand to end up with the wrist level with your left shoulder and about one shoulder-width away from the body. This results in your arm being held out at an angle of forty-five degrees, a position which ensures great strength in the elbow joint.

The right hand, meanwhile is held by the right thigh, with the palm facing backwards. It is very important that you do not simply let this hand sag down by your side; it must have some life in it.

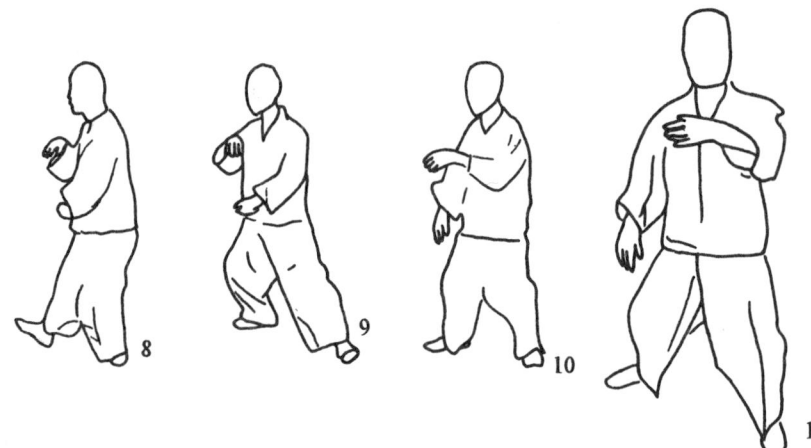

YOU LAN JUE WEI - PENG , LU , JI , AN
Grasp the Sparrow's Tail
Ward Off, Rollback, Press and Push

In this movement you once again find ways to use circles and angles, as you move forwards and backwards. Thus training the delicate sensitivity that when fully developed and applied to pushing hands will lead the opponent off-balance, without him even realising that it is happening.

In tai chi chuan great importance is placed on ensuring that the shoulders remain relaxed throughout this sequence of movements, and that the waist moves as freely and as loosely as possible. As you practise these four movements which embody the PENG (ward-off), LU (rollback), JI (press) and AN (push) principles, you will become aware of how the waist functions in initiating and carrying through every move of the upper body. The general pattern which repeats itself throughout the form is that when the waist moves forward, one or other of the arms also goes forward, and when the waist turns at least one of the arms goes with it.

Within the movements of the form are contained a number of principles which prove extremely useful in application. The first of these, PENG, describes and illustrates a kind of energy which intercepts the opponent and prevents him from closing the range too much; yet at the same time does not interfere with the movement so greatly that he is enabled to use your own force against you. In order to be efficient PENG JING must also be sensitive, so that you can "listen" and "understand" the opponent's attack.

Within the form the principles embodied in PENG are expressed in two different ways. In Left Ward-Off the right hand is kept down by the right thigh, while in Right Ward-Off the left hand comes up in a supporting role behind the right hand. In both cases attention must be paid to the hand that is not executing PENG, as without this one side of the body then becomes 'dead' and it will be easy for your opponent to knock you over.

A good starting-point for the principle LU, which is most commonly translated as rollback, is to examine it in terms of two major variations. One of which might be termed "short LU", while the other is "long LU". In both cases the principle applied must contain PENG energy, which is manifested as the potential to control the opponent's attack in any direction. In both cases the move is an intercepting one whereby the opponent's strike is met and turned to the side. In the case of "short LU" the movement is a small one whereas the "long LU" takes the opponent down and may be accompanied by a strike or lock on the elbow joint. When executing the move the waist is of vital importance and provides the motivating power. In the form the weight is shifted from the front leg to the back leg as the waist turns across the body, but the principle may also be applied with the waist turning in the other direction across the front leg and with the roles of the arms reversed. Another important point concerning the application of this principle is that the hand that is not executing the rollback is held in the ward-off position across the chest and performs a vital function. In the case of "long LU" it is this PENG hand which intercepts the opponent's strikes, uses CAI (which literally may be translated as "pluck" or pull down) to pull him down and to the side, while the other hand applies the LU against the opponent's elbow or shoulder.

The key to using "short LU" is the same as for the majority of tai chi chuan applications. The opponent must be diverted from his original intention but without being aware that this is happening until it is too late. Thus the original interception must be soft yet firm.

Another point that must be made about LU concerns the structure of the body and how it works. LU is executed with the palm facing in and the outer side of the arm facing the opponent. This is much stronger than if the palm were facing outward, and allows you to use PENG energy if your opponent pushes in against your arm. Try it both ways with a partner pushing against your arm and see for yourself which is stronger.

One of the major functions of LU is to manoeuvre your opponent into a position where he is vulnerable, and this usually occurs when he is overextended and has to withdraw. At the time that you sense this withdrawal occurring then you must move in to attack.

The process of following withdrawal with attack is exemplified in JI (or press), where you shift your weight from the back leg to the front, turn the waist, and with your forward hand applying PENG energy, you then reinforce this with the back hand joining the other, palm to palm. In order to maintain the structural strength of this posture both arms must be kept bent with the elbows down. Although in the form this movement principle is illustrated with the force being issued from the joined hands, this would be extremely difficult in a fighting situation. The principle, however, of, one force adding to another and thus creating a greater force may be used to good effect. First your front hand intercepts the opponent and then the other hand strikes. This strike may be aimed anywhere but it is most likely that the first interception will have slightly turned your opponent, opening up his side to attack. As you strike, your intercepting hand continues to apply force thus further disrupting, and ultimately destroying your opponent's stability.

In Cheng stye tai chi chuan, JI is expressed in the solo form as a movement that comes from the left hand side of the body to the right hand side in a diagonal line. This illustrates that in application this principle is best used to attack from the side.

The final section of the group of postures referred to as LAN CHI WEI (Grasp the Sparrow's Tail) is AN or push. Presented in the form as a double-handed push originating from a stance where the practitioner sits on their back leg, and then delivers the push by shifting forward onto the front leg, in fact this principle applies to any situation where both hands are placed on the opponent's body prior to delivery of an attack. But the "classics" warn that you should not use an equal amount of strength in both hands when you use AN. The reason for this is quite simple, for by only using one hand at a time the other hand is always free to follow-up. When both hands apply an equal amount of force a situation occurs which is one example of what the tai chi chuan jargon refers to as "double-weighting". In practical terms double-weighting is a situation where you have not left yourself a way out, where there is no clear distinction between YIN and YANG. If this sounds over- philosophical you can think of YIN and YANG in terms of full and empty; weight-bearing and non weight-bearing; applying strength and not applying strength; up and down, forward and backward, the list is endless. Each of these pairs may be applied to your movement and posture, and by ensuring that these opposites are always embodied in your movement you will find that you can make tai chi chuan work for you. In addition to its manifestation as a two-handed push in the solo form, AN also occurs as a single hand push in the SAN SHOU (tai chi chuan's fighting form which may be practised solo or with a partner).

Now to the form movements themselves. From Left Ward-Off sink the left hip, so adding more weight on to the left leg. As you do this let your right hand come around the waist, palm up as your left hand sinks and turns palm down so that you are holding a ball.

Then turn your waist to the right and pivot on the ball of the right foot, preparing to step out with that foot. As you step forward allow the right arm to rise up in front of you with the palm facing the chest, while the left hand turns palm down and drops slightly. As you complete the weight shift to the right leg, turn the waist to face your new front and bring the back foot around pivoting on the heel.

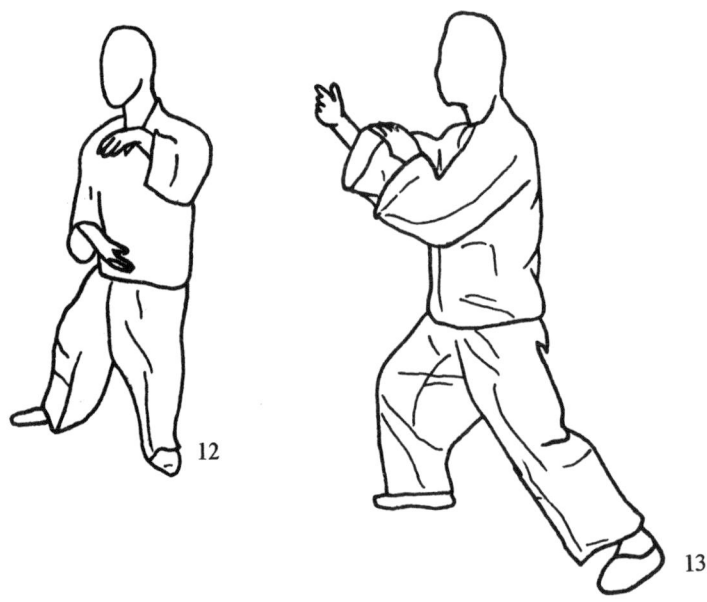

The first action you perform when moving from Ward-Off to Rollback, is the same as you have performed before you turned into the Right Ward-Off. Sink the right hip slightly and then allow the shoulders to relax and both wrists to turn slightly counter clockwise to further relax the shoulders.

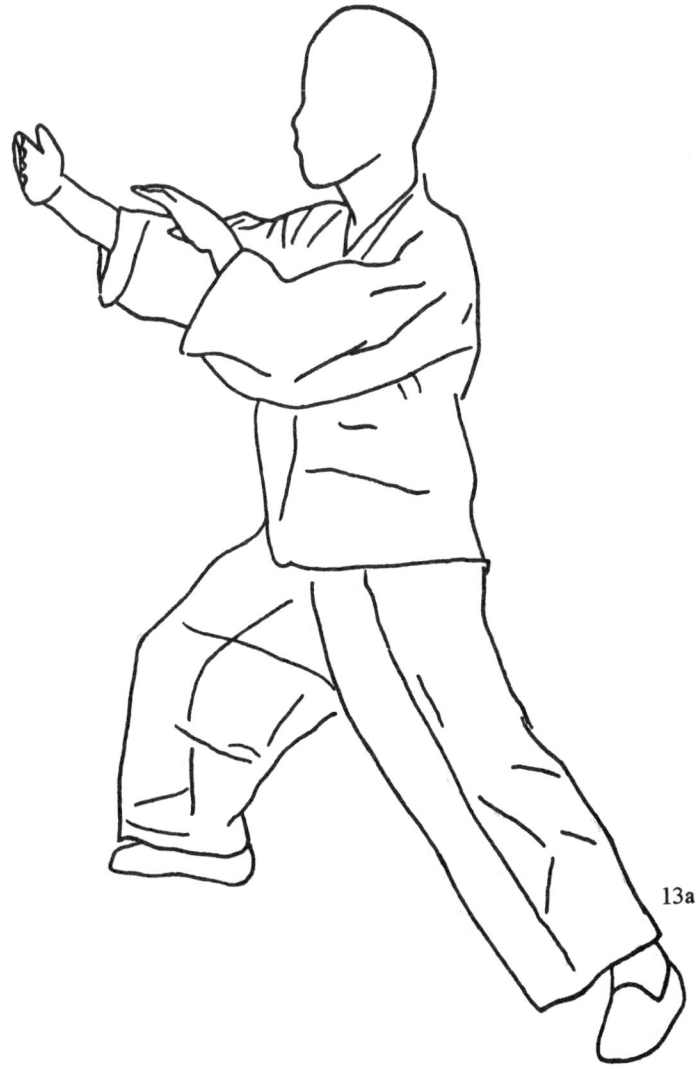

13a

Next you sink back on to the left leg, at the same time allowing the left arm to drop back across the chest into a Ward-Off position.

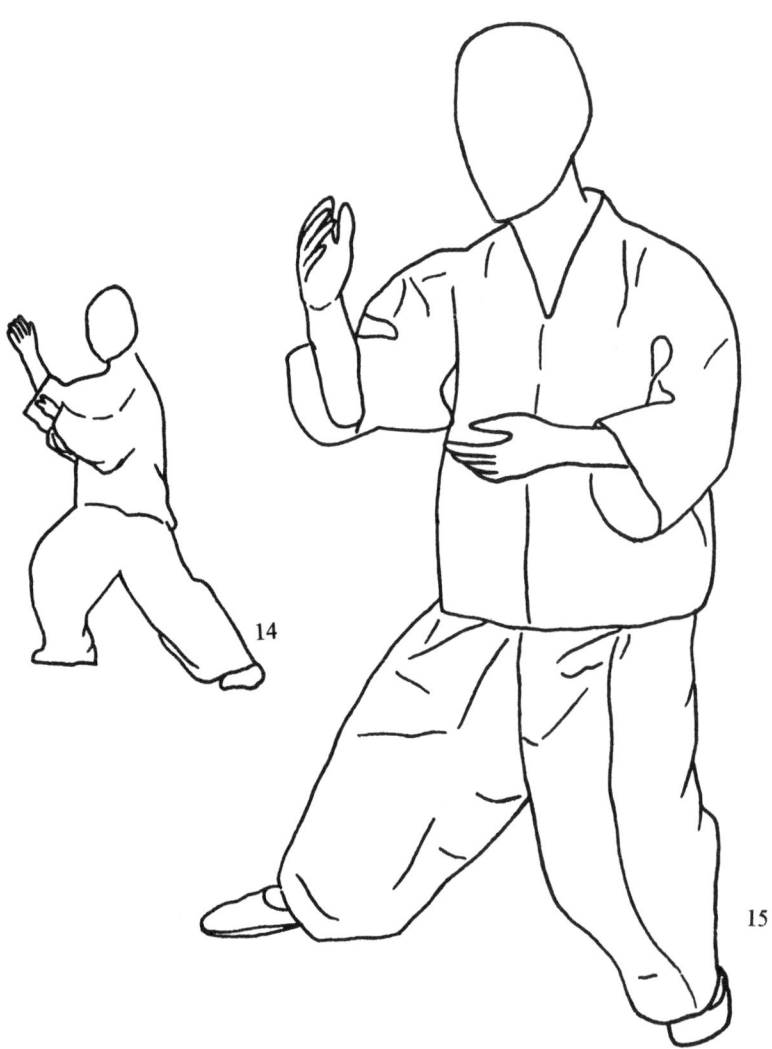

Once the root has been shifted to the back leg, start turning the waist to the left with the right arm following the action of the waist, palm facing left. When your waist has turned back as far as it can while still keeping the hips and shoulders square, allow your left hand to drop away and then turn the arm over from the elbow, making sure that you do not overstretch your shoulder joint.

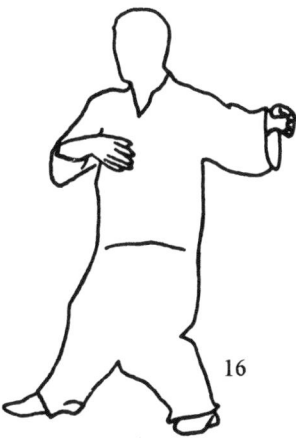

16

As the arm turns, the palm first faces up and then as your waist starts to turn to the right and the weight is shifted forward to the front foot, your left palm comes up to join the other palm in the press position.

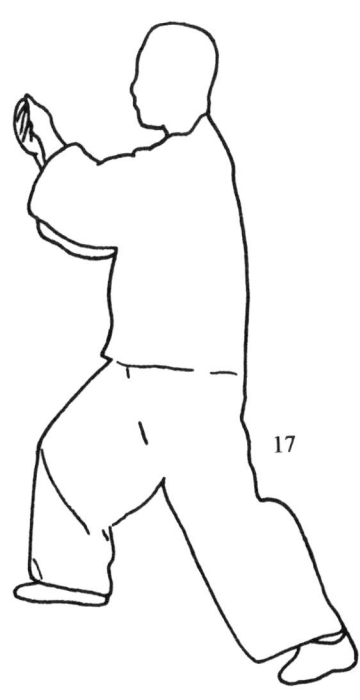

17

From here you shift your weight back on to the left leg, at the same time separating the hands, palms facing away, taking care to keep the elbows down. The hands move out until the wrists are level with your shoulders. The elbows are bent at an angle of about forty-five degrees. Then shift the weight back to the front leg, allowing the elbows to be carried forward by the momentum. This move is push. Your wrists should not go above shoulder height.

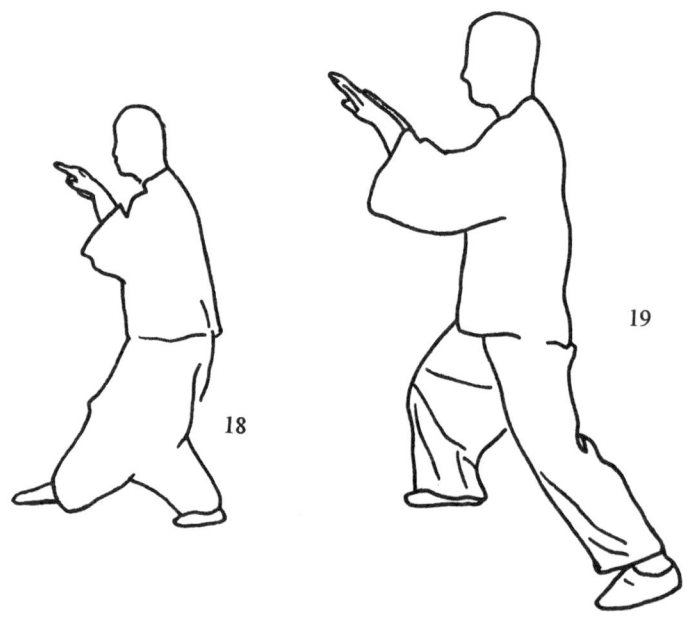

ZHUAN SHEN DIAO SHOU
Turn body and drop the hands

Although this is not a posture in itself this movement which occurs between AN and DAN BIAN embodies a number of important principles and illustrates some fundamental aspects of the practice of tai chi chuan.

First of all you sit back on the left leg allowing your arms to drop from the elbows until they parallel the floor, thus relaxing the back muscles. Then turn your waist as far as it will go to the left, keeping the arms in the same position relative to the body as they follow it around. Allow your right foot to pivot on the heel turning the toes as far as they will go to the left. Next shift your weight to the right foot, turning your waist to the right and dropping both hands so that they hold a small ball by the right hip, with the right on top.

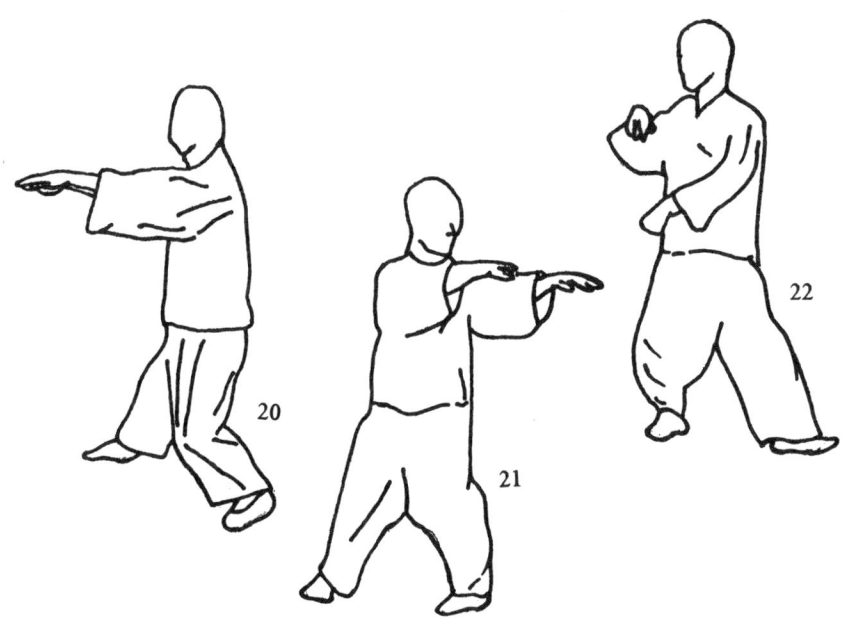

As you turn your waist and shift your weight directly after AN (turning the body or ZHUAN SHEN in Chinese) you are screwing your weight down into the ground on first one leg then the other. This is a vital part of the rooting process. By turning your waist as far as you can you promote flexibility in both the waist and the hips, thus laying the foundation for the development of power.

As your weight shifts back to the right leg your hands drop down in the movement known as DIAO SHOU. This move which can prove extremely useful in freestyle pushing hands is actually a variant of CAI (pull down) and is used to grasp and pull down your opponent's hand.

Hidden within this move, as the waist turns back to the right, is an elbow strike with the right elbow. The importance of this move lies in the fact that it occurs naturally as a result of the turning of the waist.

At this point it is worth noting that it is seldom of much use to actually perform the movements of the form as if you were hitting, kicking or performing any of the wide range of offensive and defensive techniques to be found there. For this tends to have the effect of making you tense up. Instead the form contains all of these movements and by practising in a natural and relaxed manner you allow both your body and mind to become accustomed to moving in the way designed to most efficiently maximise the power that results from total mental and physical coordination.

DAN BIAN - Single Whip

The application of the movement that is called DAN BIAN or Single Whip is actually to be found in the movement preceding the actual posture. After you have dropped your hands, and with your weight on the back leg, as you turn your waist away from the back leg, the back hand which has formed into a hook, moves out and up to the side. At the same time the front hand goes forward as the weight shifts forward on to the front leg. Then finally as the waist turns so that the hips and shoulders face forwards, the front hand turns so that the palm is facing away from the body.

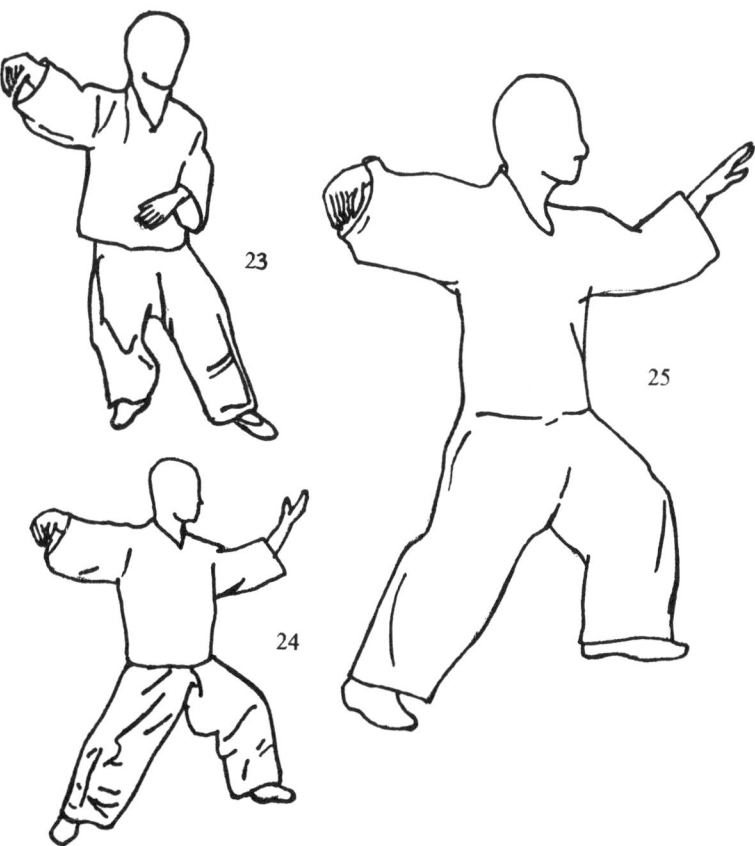

The key point in this little sequence is that, in fact, the hand that has formed a hook acts as a kind of uppercut, with the bony top of the wrist coming up to attack such "soft" targets as the bottom of the opponent's chin. This hand moves out and up because of the turning of the waist, and the more loose and relaxed this waist movement is, the more fast and powerful this tai chi chuan uppercut will be. As with many of the preceding moves, when the waist moves forward one of the hands also moves forward and when the waist turns one of the hands also turns. The final posture is an expansive one with the limbs extended and it is very important that you make every effort to relax, particularly the shoulder, elbow and wrist joints. The limb are supposed to be, according to the "classic" writings of tai chi chuan, "Straight, but not straight : bent, but not bent" !

One other common explanation for the way that this movement is performed is that the hook actually represents grasping your opponent's hand, while your other hand comes underneath his arm to strike him across the chest. The effect of this strike is augmented by your front leg being placed behind your opponent's front leg thus causing him to lose his balance. While this is one possible application it is extremely unlikely that even the most accomplished tai chi chuan practitioner would be able to carry out so complex and intricate a series of movements in the stressful and fluid situation of a fight. Instead in Zhong Ding tai chi chuan we stress the principles inherent in each movement and try to work on the infinite number of ways these principles might be applied. Repeated practice of the solo form enables these principles to become a deeply engrained part of both your physical movement and your mental attitude.

TI SHOU SHANG SHI - Lift Hands

This posture, lift hands, provides a useful illustration of the way in which small, sometimes barely, discernible, movements contain vital lessons. From DAN BIAN you turn your waist to the right. This has the effect of screwing down the weight on to the left leg. At the same time both arms open slightly and the shoulders drop downwards, which enables them to relax. The back leg is then pulled back in towards the left leg. Again, as with the preceding arm and shoulder move, this move is just enough to relax the right hip and the foot does not have to come right in to the other leg. As the right hip relaxes, the right leg then moves out directly to the right, ending up on the right heel. Simultaneously both arms drop and then raise with the right arm forward thus putting the whole of the right side forward. The left hand is level with the right elbow. In Zhong Ding tai chi chuan in both this posture and SHOU HUI PIPA, which is similar in appearance, the hands are kept shoulder-width apart with the elbows out and naturally hanging down to further promote relaxation.

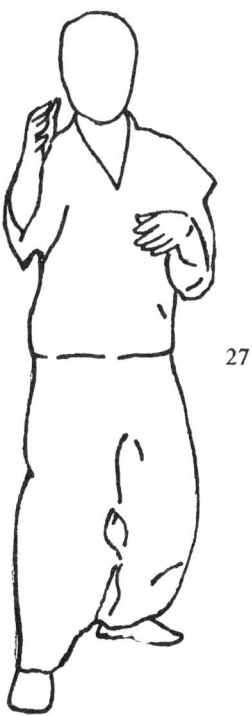

27

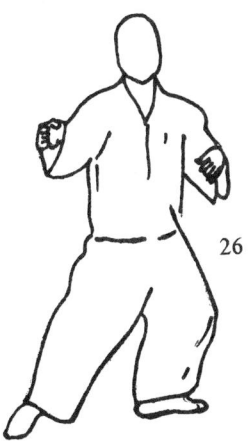

26

This small "in-out" leg movement of the right leg in fact simulates a tai chi chuan kicking motion, as the hip joint moves through the same range of motion required of it when kicking, with the motivating power coming from the turning of the waist. The small upward movement of the arms also illustrates one of the basic responses the tai chi chuan practitioner has to an attack. Reflexively lifting the hands both disrupts the opponent's attack and provides you with an opening. Because we are constantly lifting up our arms and working against gravity in our daily lives this action is very natural. Professor Cheng Man Ching, the founder of our system of tai chi chuan, recommends static practice of this posture to develop the strength of the legs, while his teacher Yang Cheng Fu reportedly practised DAN BIAN for expansive power, and TI SHOU SHANG SHI, for contracting power. Once you are in this posture you must pay careful attention to relaxing both the hips and the shoulders. In order to ensure that the front leg remains relaxed you must check that the toes are not raised too high.

KAO - Shoulder strike

KAO is one of the eight movement principles that are repeated throughout the form. Its main application is as a shoulder strike but it also contains ZHOU, or elbow strike. This occurs either as the right leg steps out before the shoulder strike or after the shoulder strike if you have to readjust your range from the opponents or withdraw. At the end of the move prior to stepping out into the next move you turn your waist to the right. This illustrates the concept of "swing and movement" and also points out how this move may be used in pushing hands. For if the initial shoulder strike fails, by turning your waist to, in the case of the form, the right side, you disrupt the opponent's balance enough to make him pull back, you may then apply a technique that works in the other direction. This is a key principle in tai chi chuan, which works primarily as a counter-attacking art, whereby you make use of your opponent's mistakes or weaknesses. Of course, if your opponent appears to have no weaknesses, you must put him in a position where he gives you the opportunity that you need. So it is that you may have to attack first.

Bring in the right foot as you drop both hands so that the right hand rests on the lower abdomen and the left hand rests on the left thigh. The legs hang naturally, slightly open.

Then step forward again with the right foot. As the weight shifts the momentum carries your right elbow slightly forward, with your palm turned up. This move approximates to an elbow strike. Your rear, left hand goes on to rest on the inside of the right elbow. As you arrive in the posture you adjust the back foot and right at the very end you turn the waist to the right.

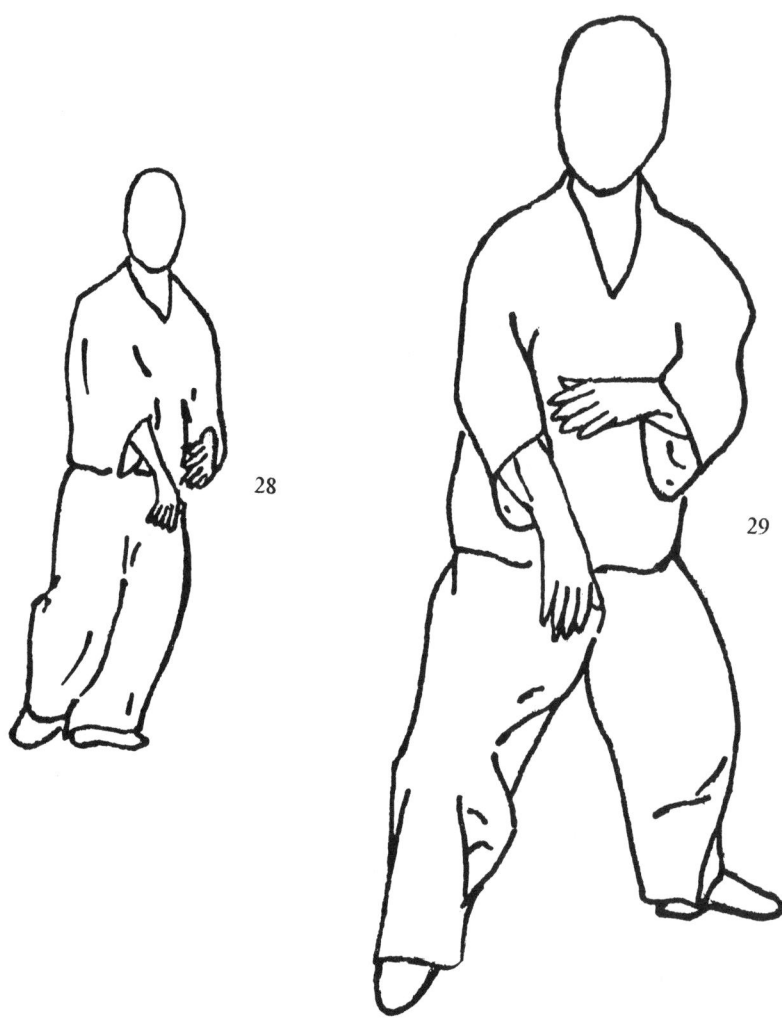

BAI HE LIANG CHI
White Crane Spreads Its Wings

As the name suggests White Crane Spreads Its Wings is an expansive gesture, where you feel as if your arms are the wings of a large bird. Contained within this posture are a number of important manifestations of the tai chi chuan principles. While the weight is sunk on the right leg, the right hand is held high thus creating a balance of YIN and YANG. In the same way while the left leg is held with only a fraction of the weight resting on the toes, and therefore in tai chi chuan terms is empty, it is the left hand that is, in application terms, doing the bulk of the work. This is because the bottom hand is deflecting a punch or strike. As it deflects, this hand must also disrupt your opponent's balance enough to allow you to exploit the weakness you have created. Having created this opening your right hand may be used to strike the opponent's face or upper body. The principle being applied here is that of engaging the opponent low and then attacking high, or vice-versa. This again corresponds with YIN-YANG theory. In practical terms you are trying to give the opponent pain in one area so that you can inflict more pain in another area. The fact is that human beings can become very quickly accustomed to pain in one particular area, therefore you strive to keep them both mentally and physically off-balance by constantly changing your target areas.

Because the right hand is held high there is a tendency for the right shoulder to become tense and you must keep it relaxed. As with the majority of the tai chi chuan postures the hips and shoulders form a rectangle. There is also a possibility with any posture that involves the majority of the weight being placed on the back leg, that the front leg can be used to kick. It must be remembered, however, that tai chi chuan kicks work at close range, and you should endeavour never to kick unless you have a hold on some part of the opponent's anatomy. In Tai Chi Chuan this is described as kicking when you have three legs on the ground : one of your own and two of your opponent's.

From the previous move turn the waist to the right then allow the waist to unwind to the left. This has the effect of bringing the back foot in and then moving it out again in a semi-circular action with the toes pointing to what is now your front. The heel is up off the ground as the weight stays on the right leg. As the waist turns the right hand comes up across the right side of the chest with the palm turning to face upwards and out away from the body. The arm remains bent. At the same time the left arm comes down and brushes the left knee.

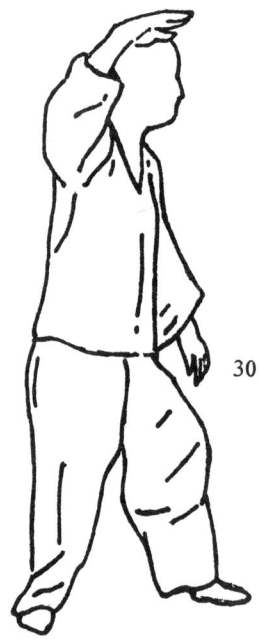

30

LOU CHI AO BU
Brush Knee Twist Step

The title of this movement Brush Knee and Twist Step so called because the opposite arm and leg are forward, shows the importance of the hand that appears to be doing the least work, for it refers to the bottom hand and not the one that is performing a striking action.

As you move into this posture you learn an important lesson about the connection between the hand and foot. If you are moving into a left stance, as the left foot touches down, the right hand relaxes at the wrist and sinks down by the right ear, having risen up in a circle at the right diagonal rear. Then as the waist turns and the weight is shifted forward onto the left leg, the right hand raises as it is pushed forward, until it is once again in line with the rest of the forearm. Meanwhile the left hand has "brushed" around the left knee. In application this would parry a low kick or punch so opening up the opponent to the right palm strike.

The fact that the right wrist sinks as the left ankle relaxes illustrates the connection between the wrist and the ankle, and also shows the cross-connection between the left hand and the right foot and vice-versa which is found in so many of the movements of the form.

This brush knee twist step posture is repeated, several times throughout the form, and this in itself points out the importance of this movement. Certainly it is extremely effective as a fighting technique and is used in a large number of Chinese martial arts other than Tai Chi. Indeed a few years ago I attended a Chinese martial arts tournament at which one particular school used this technique almost to the exclusion of any other. They were highly successful, winning three separate weight categories.

In order to successfully apply this move you must ensure that the waist provides the momentum to carry around the relaxed and consequently heavy arms. In this way your parrying arm will also damage the opponent's limb, momentarily distracting him from your impending palm attack. As with many other Tai Chi hand strikes, the fingers touch softly to ascertain the nature of the resistance you are likely to encounter, and then the palm smashes in. This is, of course, a practical example of the "ting jing" or listenning energy of the art. All this means in layman's terms is that you first try to feel out the opponent's weak spots so that you can disrupt his balance before you hit him, thus maximising the effect of your attack.

From White Crane Spreads its Wings, turn your waist to the right and allow the right arm to drop down so that both hands form the bear posture to the right.

Next step out with the left foot into a front stance as the right arm turns up, palm upwards and then folds at the elbow so that as the left foot is put down the right hand folds at the wrist to sink down by the ear. Then as you shift the weight to the front foot the left hand brushes the knee and the right hand extends forward to execute a palm strike at shoulder height.

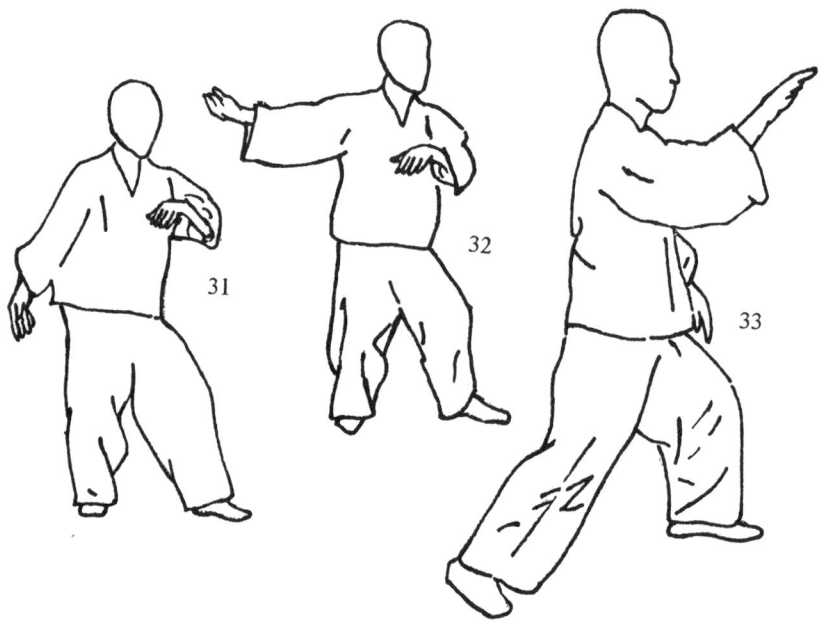

SHOU HUI PIPA
Strum the Lute

In Zhong Ding Tai Chi Chuan this movement is very similar to lift hands, the only difference being that the hands are not held so high.

In moving into this posture you practise a type of movement that will stand you in good stead when you come to practise pushing hands or fighting skills.

As you move from Brush Knee Twist Step, the waist turns slightly to the left thus placing the weight even more solidly over the left leg. This has the effect of releasing the back (right) leg so that it can take half a step forward, to be placed down at approximately right angles to the front foot. As it is put down the right hand drops slightly and the left hand rises up. At the same time the left leg is lifted up, brought in slightly and finally put down with the weight resting on the heel and the toes raised off the ground a little. It is important, from the point of view of relaxation, that the front knee remains bent.

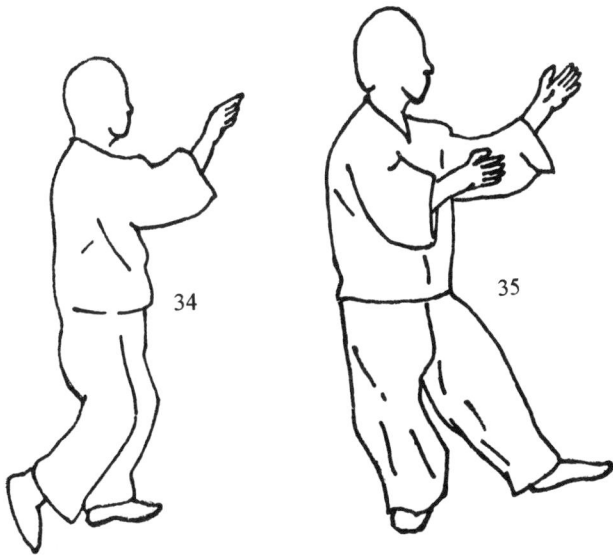

34

35

As with Lift Hands the wrists are kept shoulder-width apart with the elbow slightly out so that the chest may be as relaxed as possible.

The classical interpretation of this movement is that it is a double-handed arm break, with the hand nearest your body pushing down on the opponent's wrist, while the other hand pushes against the elbow joint. That this is not clearly seen in the Zhong Ding Tai Chi Chuan form is a reflection of the major emphasis on relaxation at this stage of the training process.

The importance of the half step up taken by the rear leg is that it is a key form of movement in pushing hands and fighting. The movement of the rear leg adds impetus to the attack, putting the full weight of the body behind your move. To disguise the build-up of your strength, you must take care that your arms remain relaxed, and the shoulders in particular must not become tense and rigid. This becomes of crucial importance when practising pushing hands, because unless you can so disguise your leg manoeuvres your opponent will always be able to use listening energy or "ting jing" to anticipate and thwart your moves.

LOU XI AO BU

Repeat the moves described above.

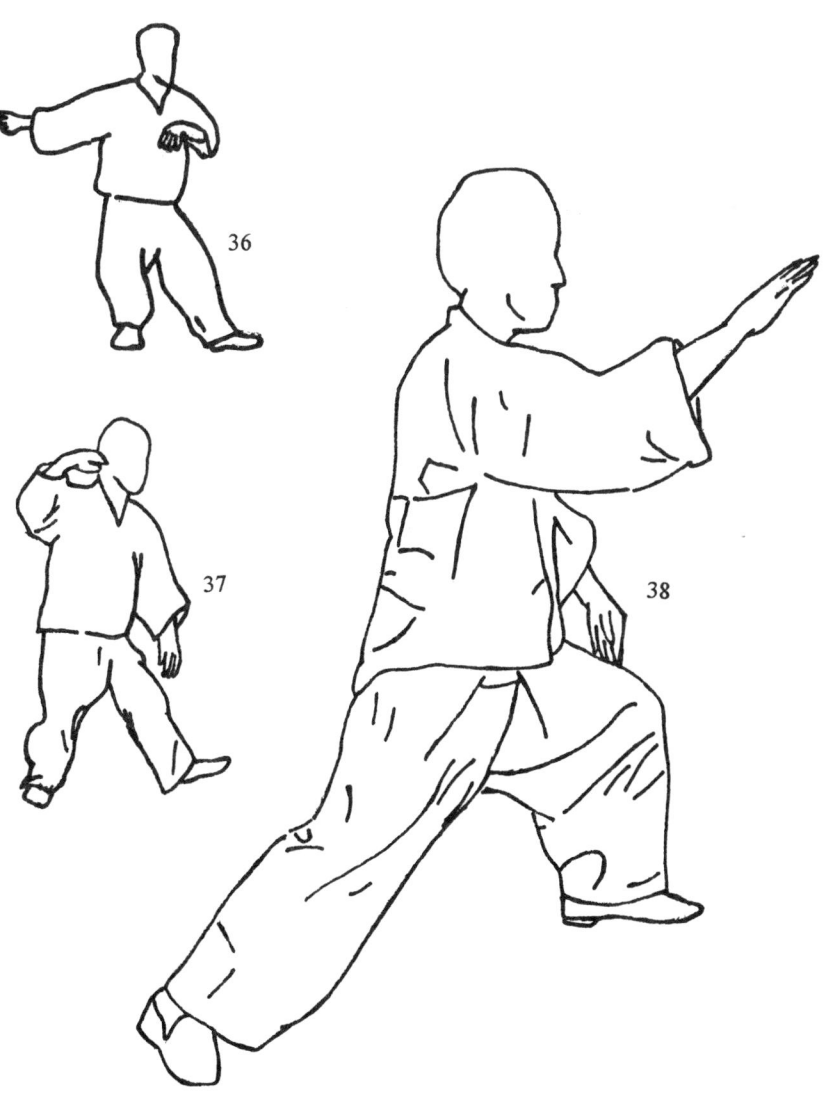

JING BU BAN LAN CHUI
Step Forward, Move, Parry, Punch

From Brush Knee Twist Step you sit back onto the right leg while turning the waist to the left. As you do so the shoulders relax thus causing the hands to turn in slightly so that the palms are facing each other. The effect of turning the waist to the left is that the left foot turns out to approximately forty-five degrees; the weight is then shifted on to it. The waist then starts to turn to the right and the right foot comes slightly in and then turns out to be placed in front of the left foot and turned out to ninety degrees. As this happens the right hand which has formed a fist as the weight was shifted to the left foot, moves up and over in a clockwise vertical action, executing what is in effect a small backfist action, until it rests on the right hip; while the left hand is extended in front of the body with the open palm facing to the right. The left foot then steps forward and as the weight is transferred to it, the left hand parries over and down. The waist is then turned to face front thus causing the right hand to punch forward with the fist held in a vertical position and the open left hand rests palm down, with the fingers lightly touching the right elbow region.

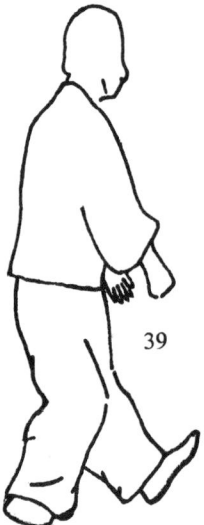

39

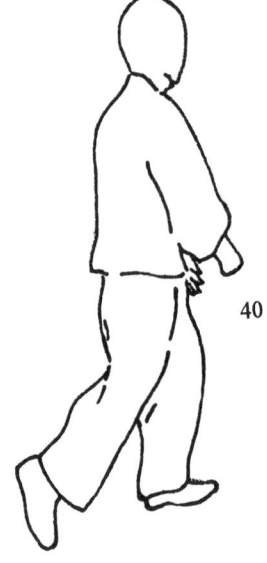

40

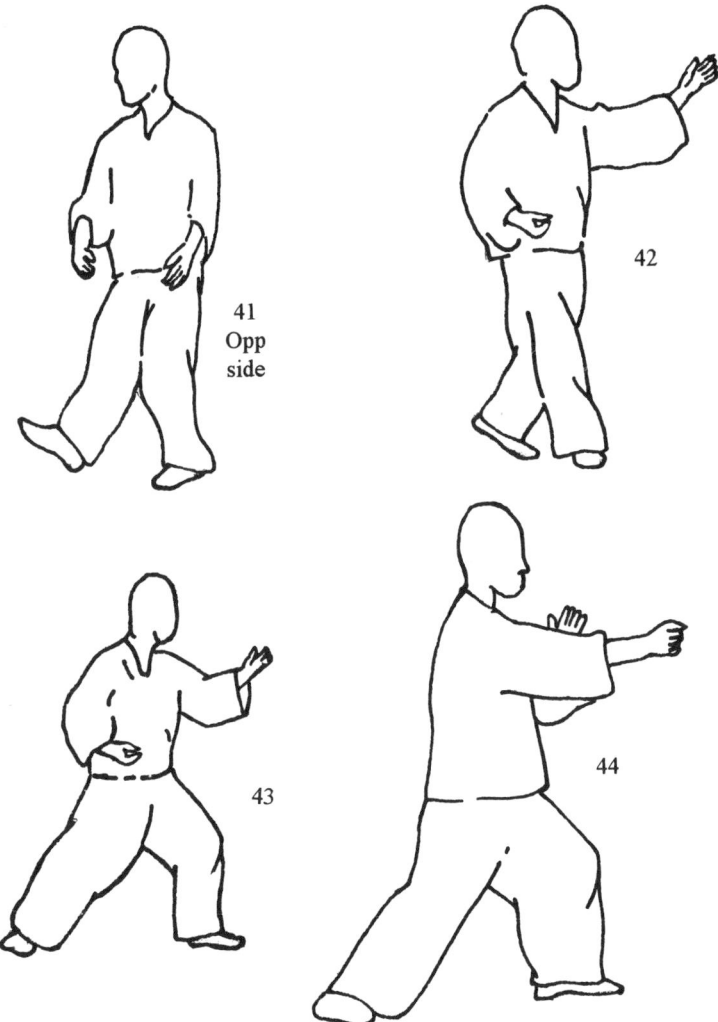

41
Opp
side

42

43

44

In this technique you will practise using your whole body with the power emanating from the waist. This teaches you to maximise your own physical potential. So that if, for example, your wrist was being held, rather than just using your arm to try to escape, you instead turn your waist first one way and then the other, in effect shaking off, your attacker and then following your opponent's retreating movement with your own attack. Note that the fist attack is aimed at the soft target area of the lower abdomen, from the solar plexus down to the groin.

RUFENG SIBI
As If Closing a Door

In this movement, from the previous posture, you sit back on to the right leg. As you do so the left hand turns so that it is almost palm up underneath the right arm and the right hand is pulled back over the top of the other arm. The right arm folds in slightly towards the left, bending at the elbow. As you finally arrive back as far as you can comfortably go both arms cross and then open out into the same position as in AN, which movement you then execute.

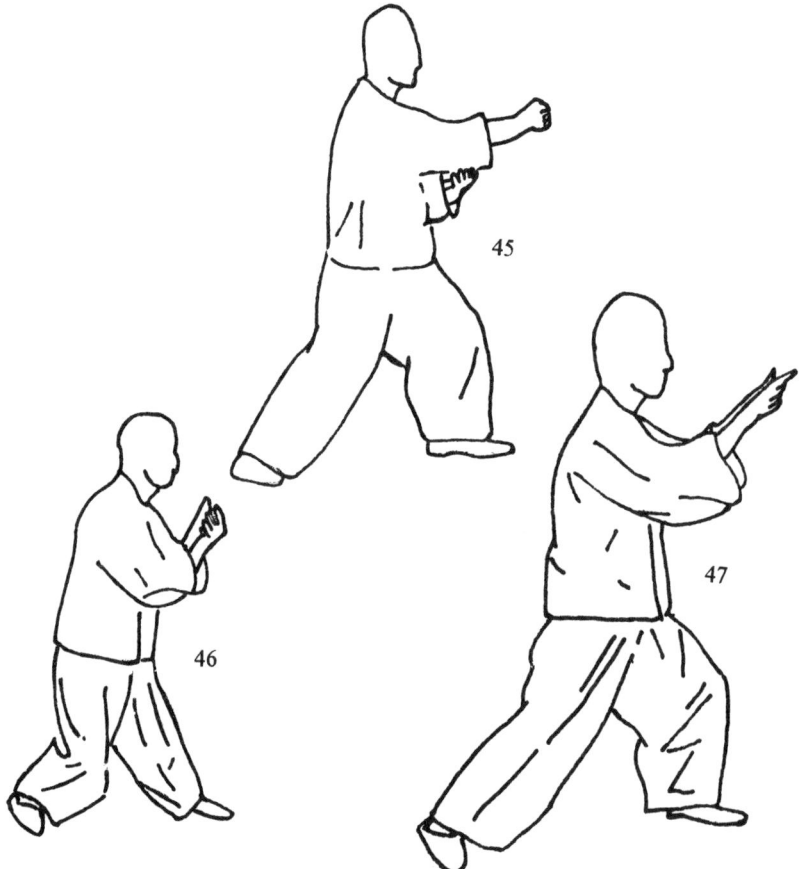

The most obvious reason for the name of this posture is that you appear to be offering your opponent an ideal opportunity, when you sit on your leg and cross your arms. But that this is only "apparent" is shown by the way in which the left arm comes underneath and actually opens up the other person to attack.

This movement is of vital importance to you when you start practising freestyle pushing hands. It enables you to use an opponent's attack to your advantage and to learn how to snatch victory from the jaws of defeat.

SHIZI SHOU - Cross Hands

From the push at the end of the previous move, you sit back on to the right leg, turning the waist to face the right and pulling the left foot around, pivoting on the heel until the toes face your right. At the same time the arms first sink until the forearms are parallel with the floor, then when you have turned, the arms open up, palms facing outwards, elbows sunk.

The right foot pivots on the toes, until it is also facing the right. By now your hands are below waist level with the palms facing inwards. Next your right foot steps back so that it is level with the left foot at shoulder width distance. At the same time the hands come up to cross in front of your chest with the right hand underneath the left, both palms facing in.

When you are in the final posture your weight returns to the left leg even though it appears to be in the middle.

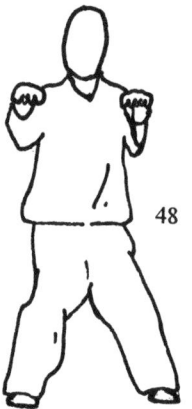
48

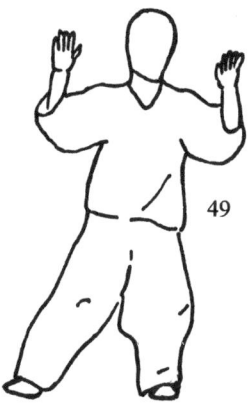
49

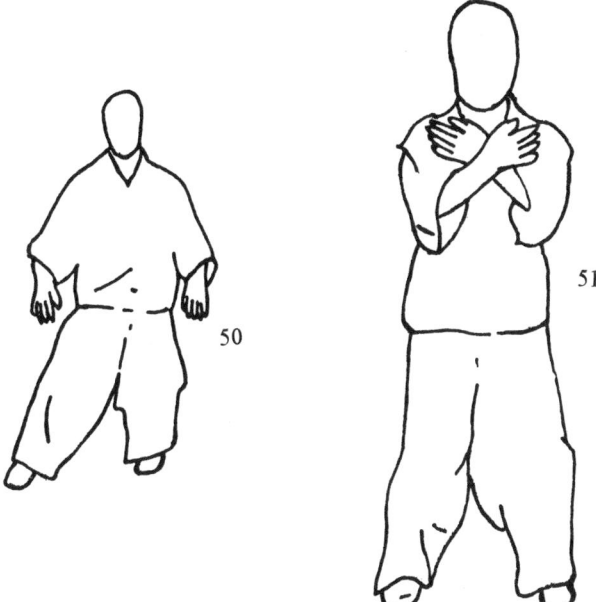

Like the previous move, Cross Hands teaches you much about diverting an opponent's attack, when practising pushing hands. For this teaches you how to bring one arm under the other to divert the opponent's push and turn it into an offensive move of your own.

BAO HU GUI SHAN
Embrace Tiger, Return To Mountain

In the previous posture your right wrist should have been holding up the left one and what you do next is turn the waist slightly to the left and at the same time allow the right hand to gently drop away, which, in turn, causes the left hand to drop down and to the left. Both hands then end up palms facing in towards your body and equidistant either side of the left thigh.

Now that you have stored up weight in your left leg, turn the waist to the right allowing the right hand to move out and around the right leg in a "Brush Knee" motion, as the right leg steps out to the right rear. At the same time the left hand turns palm up and comes over in a move very closely resembling the upper arm movement in "Brush Knee Twist Step". All of the movements are initiated from, and motivated by the waist which turns the back foot around to face forty-five degrees. In the final posture the right hand turns to face palm up and the left arm is at an angle across the body, these constituting the main differences from the "Brush Knee Twist Step" posture.

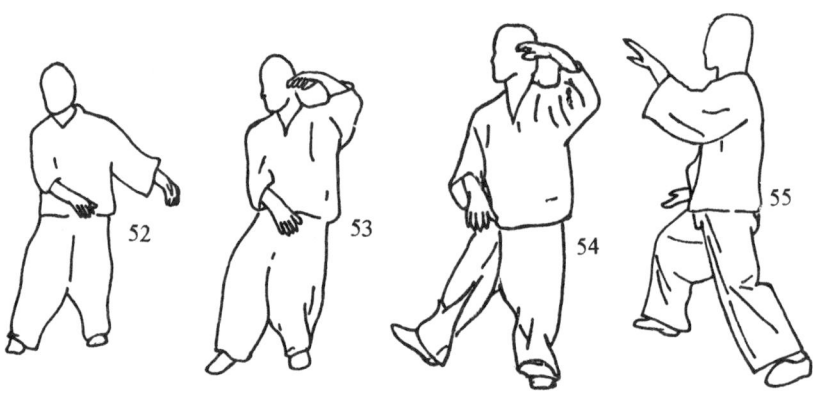

52   53   54   55

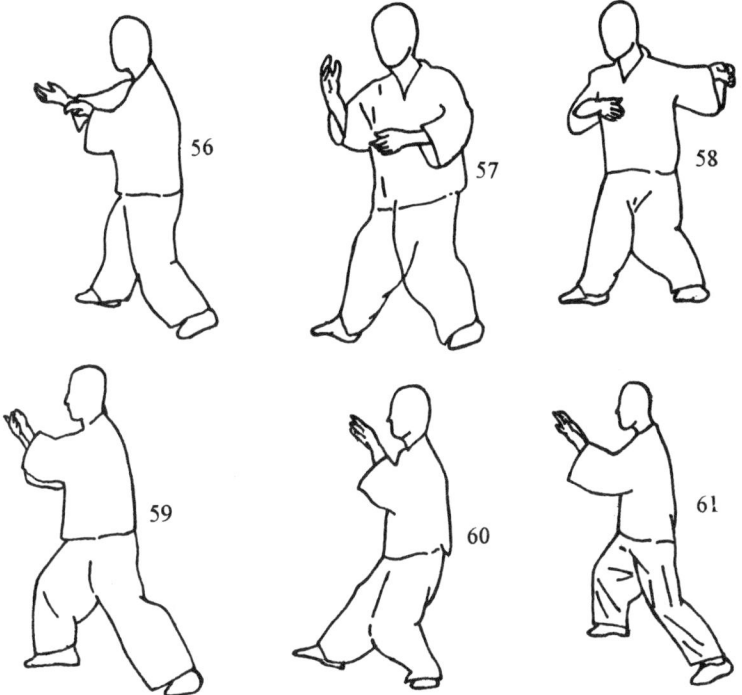

This movement illustrates the power generated by turning of the waist, and the way in which the arms, naturally following the action of the waist express the strength of the body rather than just relying on their own strength in isolation.

From your front stance sit back into the back leg, raising your right hand as you do so, and allowing your left hand to drop down naturally until it is in a ward-off position across your chest. You will find it necessary as you raise your right arm and lower your left arm to adjust the wrists slightly. The right hand rotates anti-clockwise until the palm is facing the left, while the left hand also turns anti-clockwise until the palm is facing your chest. This rotation allows the shoulders to sink and relax.

From here you follow the instructions for LU, JI and AN.

XIE DAN BIAN
Diagonal Single Whip

After AN you sit back as you have done previously and then move through all the movements exactly as if you were going to perform the ordinary Single Whip. But when your weight is on the right leg, the right hand paw already extended, instead of stepping out to the front you step to the diagonal. (See diagram). Again you must pay attention to the way that as the weight is transferred to the front leg the arm is raised with the hand only turning as the waist is turned. This is a vitally important lesson of the solo form; namely natural movement so that you learn to put your whole body into any technique.

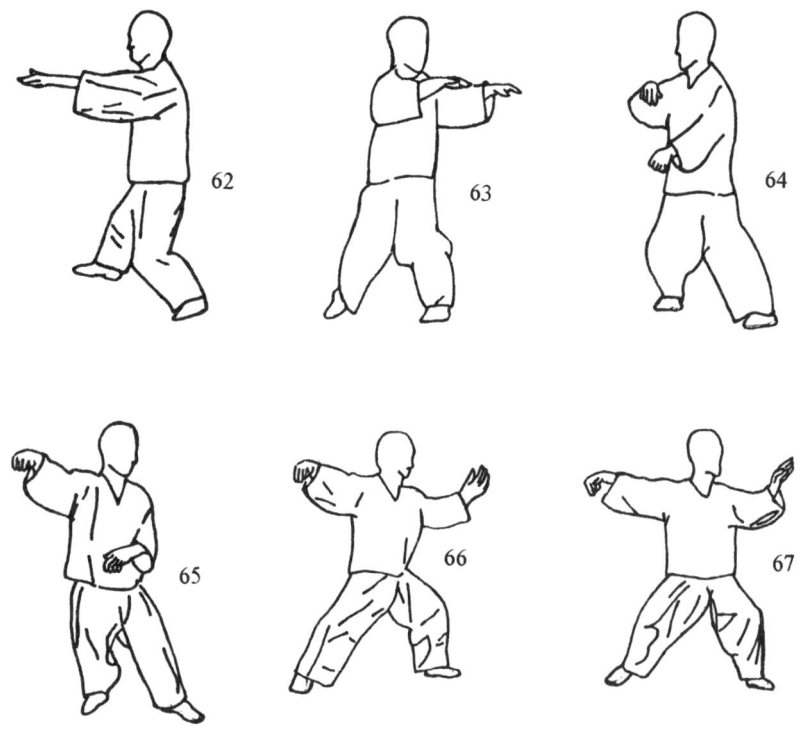

ZHOU DI KAN CHUI
Fist Under Elbow

Moving into this posture enables you to learn how to shift the weight from one leg to another and then back. This skill is vital in pushing hands and also in the development of effective fighting skills. For this enables you to quickly change your body position while still remaining in a position from which you could launch an effective attack.

From the previous posture you shift your weight back into the right leg, at the same time opening up the right hand and dropping both arms slightly in order to enable the shoulders to relax. The action of the waist moving back pulls the left leg back, lifting it off the floor and placing it down slightly to the left and to the rear of its previous position. The foot faces forward and your weight is then shifted on to it. Next you bring your foot up until it is level with the other one and about the width of your shoulders away from it. You then place it down at the same time turning your waist towards the left. This will bring your right foot around slightly. Placing your weight on the right foot, carry on your waist movement to the left allowing your left foot, to pivot around the toes. By now your right arm has moved around to a position in line with your right side as your hips face slightly diagonally to the left. At this point your left hand starts to drop towards your left hip from where it moves in a scooping up action, rather like a gunfighter scooping a gun out of a holster, and then up to your front ending up with the hand level with your left shoulder, palm facing to the right, elbow hanging down. While your left hand is executing its scooping, rising action your hips turn clockwise until they are facing directly forwards and the right arm continues its circling to the left, coming in with the forearm across the body. Finally the right hand forms into a fist with the thumb up, under the left elbow. Remember to keep a small space under both armpits so that the move uses the whole body.

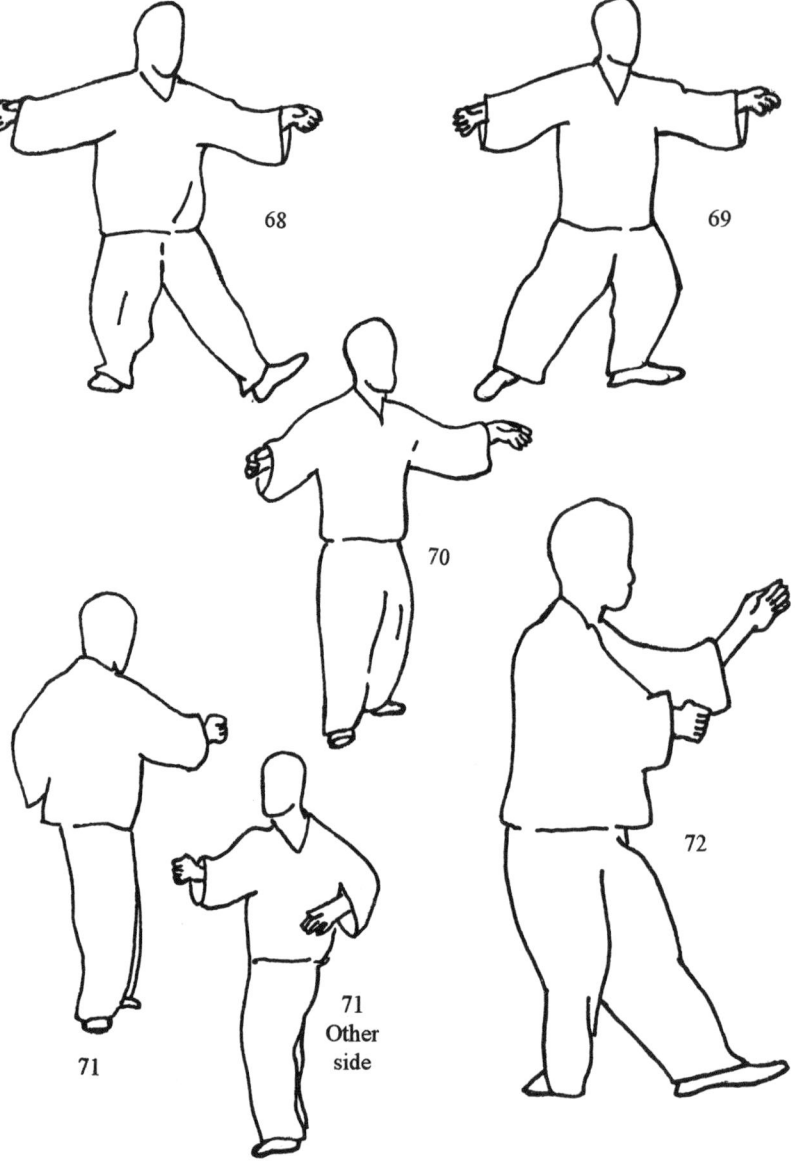

68

69

70

71

71
Other
side

72

There are various approaches to the application of this move. One story being that it was one of the "hidden" moves by which Yang Luchan hoped to prevent his Manchu employers from learning the real secrets of tai chi. The story goes that the whole move involves stepping forwards with the front foot and simultaneously parrying with the front arm while punching with the other. Now this is hardly a devastatingly secret attack and the Manchus would have to have been pretty stupid not to be able to work that move out. Couple that with the fact that Yang Luchan was teaching the Imperial Guard who would all be tried and tested combat veterans and therefore no slouches when it came to determining what would work and what wouldn't, the story seems fairly implausible.

A far more likely and effective application of this move is the use of the left hand as a parry, which once having located the opponent's arm is then used as an aiming point for a strike to the limb by the other arm.

DAO NIAN HOU
Step Back Repulse Monkey

This move embodies the movements of one of the five animals of Tai Chi, the monkey. In the closely coordinated movements of hands and feet we find the tai chi version of the scuttling backward steps of a monkey moving away from danger as he looks for an opening to attack before scampering away again out of harm's way.

The move is of fundamental importance in teaching you how to turn retreat into advance and how to find the right distance to effectively apply your tai chi if crowded by an opponent.

In order to learn the correct body mechanics of the movement we break it down into three parts and although this might seem mechanical at first, with time and practice you will soon get the flow without missing any of the vital points.

From the previous movement you turn your waist to the right allowing the left hand to extend out naturally to your front. At the same time the right hand drops down, moving in a semicircle down to the right hip and then rising up, palm up, until it is at shoulder height, and out to the right rear diagonal.

The position of the arms is now symmetrical with the hips facing the right diagonal, arms outstretched but elbows down, left palm down and right palm up. The chest is kept rounded so that the shoulders are not pulled back and tight; a good indicator of whether your arm position is correct is that with your head held naturally and facing the same direction as your hips, you should be able to see the fingers of both hands. This is an important method for training your all-round visual awareness and of exercising your peripheral vision which is a vital component of effective fighting skills.

The second part of the movement consists of turning the hips anti-clockwise, back to face front. At the same time the left hand turns palm-up, sinking slightly at the elbow, while the right arm bends at the elbow, ending up palm down by the right ear, as in the movement Brush Knee Twist Step.

The final part of the movement starts with the left foot which has been held with the weight on the heel, stepping directly back, and placing it down, toes first. The weight is then transferred back on to the left leg, rolling the foot down from toe to heel. As the weight is transferred, the left hand comes down to rest on the left hip, palm up; while the right hand pushes out to end up at shoulder height palm facing away. For the final part of this movement you turn the right foot on the heel until the toes are pointing forward. This adjustment will be unnecessary in the next two repetitions of the movement because your feet remain parallel, as if resting on railway lines.

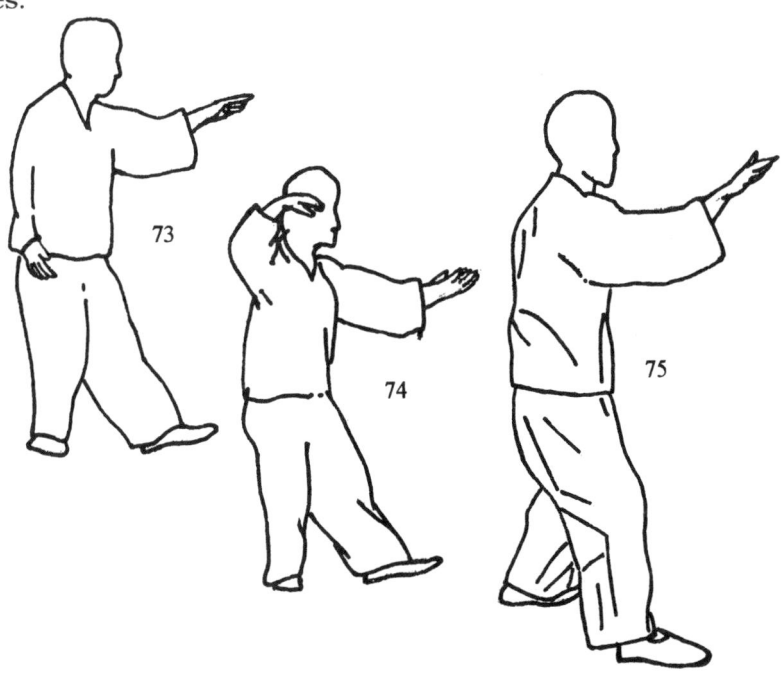

How wide the stance is depends on your size and body shape, but as a general rule it varies between half-shoulder and shoulder-width apart with the length being more or less the same. You must remember to keep the front knee bent.

This move, in its three parts, is then executed twice more, ending up with the right leg forward in the final posture.

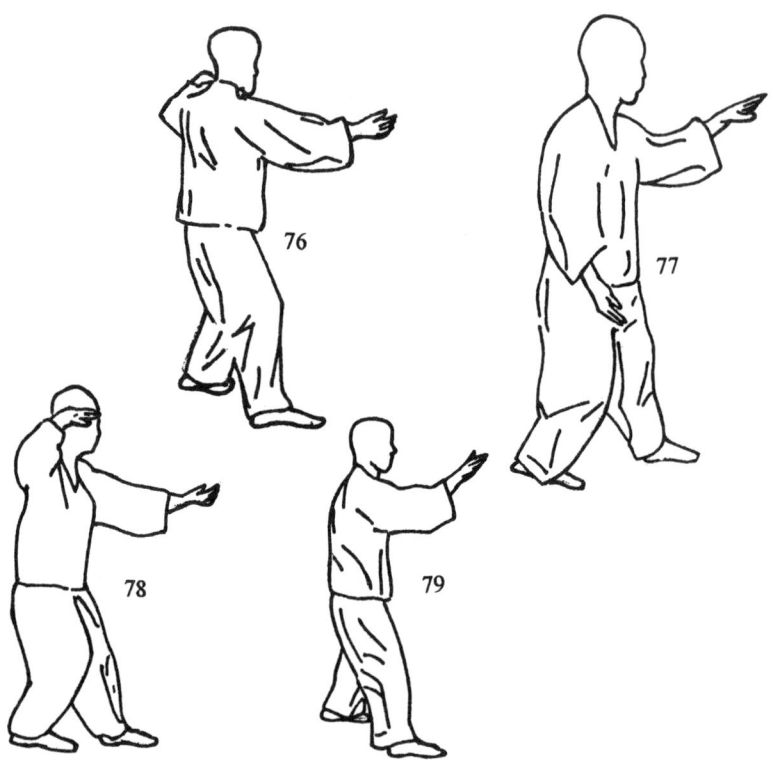

Where DAO NIAN HOU as practised in the Cheng style differs from that of the traditional Yang style is in the positioning of the back foot. In the latter it is placed at forty-five degrees while in Cheng style it faces directly forward as described above. There are a number of reasons for this.

Firstly as Cheng Man Ching points out in his writings, by adopting this foot position the exponent ensures that his back remains erect, his backside does not stick out and therefore according to Chinese medical theory his qi is able to circulate freely. In more down-to-earth physiological terms the spine is enabled to hang naturally with all the accompanying postural benefits.

Secondly by moving back in such a fashion you are training yourself, should you have to face an opponent who forces you back two or more steps, to always be in a position to counter. You can try this for yourself. First attempt to move rapidly backwards, turning out your back foot to forty-five degrees as in the Yang style version; then try it with the feet pointing forward. The major difference that you will notice is that in the former method you are prone to losing your balance and falling over backwards. In the latter form of movement your upper body always feels as if it wants to fall forward thus giving you the ability to swiftly change retreat into advance.

The third reason for practising Step Back Repulse Monkey in this way is to train flexibility in the ankles; a vital step if you are to develop the ability to use explosive force by pushing off the ground. A flexible ankle enables you to, in a paraphrase of the classics, to transmit power from the feet, to be controlled by the waist and expressed in the fingers.

For all of these reasons it is an extremely good idea to practice DAO NIAN HOU in isolation, repeating the moves over and over again until they feel stable and natural.

Another important reason for practising this move is that the upper body movements enable you, if entering into a clinch situation with your opponent, to use one arm as a lever against his body while you push off, stepping back to give yourself the space you need to strike with the other hand. Thus DAO NIAN HOU is an important tool for maintaining correct distance.

XIE FEI SHI
Diagonal Flying

This movement embodies the principle of LIE or " splitting" whereby one force is taken in one direction while force is exerted in another.

In this case the move consists of a parrying or pulling down action combined with a strike upward and in a diagonal direction.

From the last movement you turn your waist to the left, dropping the right hand to waist height and allowing the left to move out following the movement of the body, until both hands are held in the "bear" position, palms facing each other. Next you turn your waist to the right, allowing the hands to follow and hold a ball with the left hand on top. This waist movement is then carried down to the right leg which pivots slightly on the heel and then steps out to the right diagonal.

As you shift the weight forward on to the right leg, the right arm comes up inside the left arm and is then extended out with the hand at shoulder height, palm up. At the same time the left hand drops down to end up palm facing slightly down, by the left thigh.

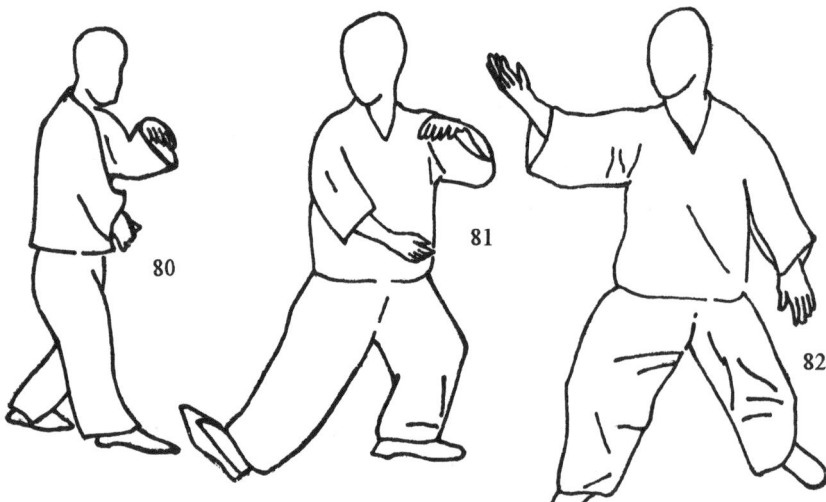

So it is that the right hand has struck to the opponent's neck or face, while the left hand has smothered, grasped or parried the incoming attack.

While doing this move take care that you keep the right hip relaxed prior to stepping out, otherwise you will find that the movement becomes clumsy.

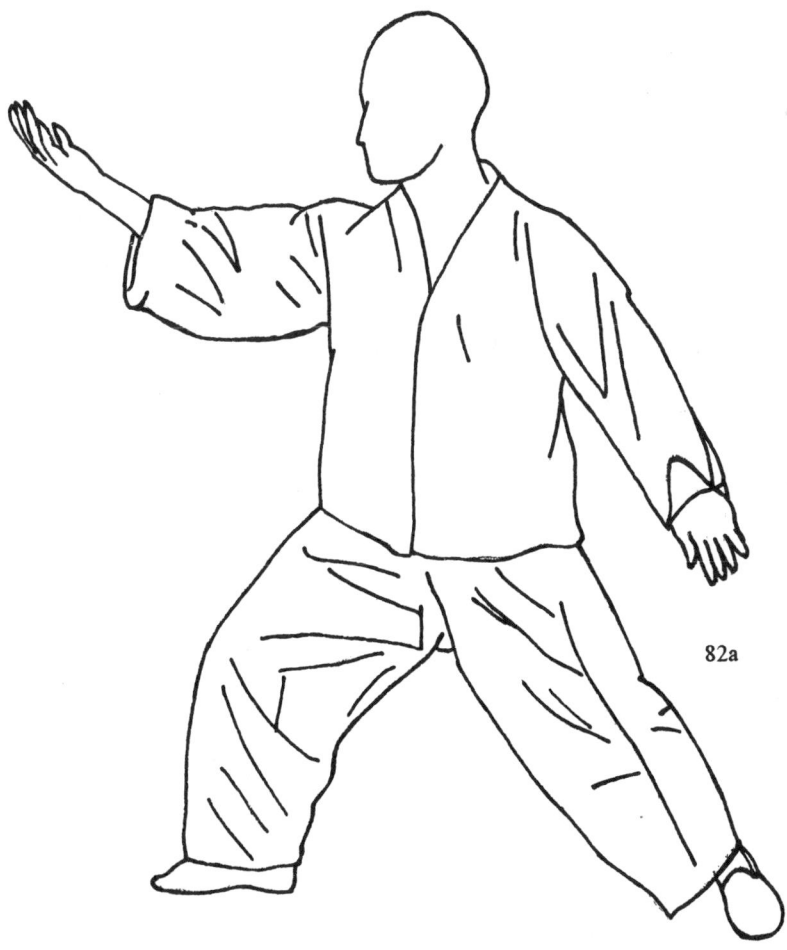

82a

YUN SHOU
Cloud Hands

When practising YUN SHOU you learn how to use the waist to provide total body power. These powerful waist movements are typical of the action of the bear and so it is that this posture is often described as embodying the characteristic movements of the bear.

From the preceding posture turn the waist slightly to the right allowing the right hand to turn palm down, dropping the elbow slightly, while the left hand comes around at waist level and turns palm up. Thus your hands end up holding a ball to your right diagonal.

The turning of your waist brings up the left leg, taking the weight off the heel first and bringing it up until it is on a line with the right foot and about one and a half shoulder-widths away from it.

Next you start to shift your weight on to the left leg. As you do so the left hand slowly comes up in a ward-off position across your chest, palm in. The right hand drops down and comes across the body at waist height also with the palm facing in. Meanwhile your waist continues turning to the left until all the weight is on the left foot. As the waist completes its turn the right foot pivots on the heel so that the toes face forward. Then with both hands holding a ball to the left, left hand on top, the right foot steps across to end up a shoulder-width away from the left.

From here start to shift the weight to the right leg and simultaneously let the left hand drop. As your waist turns to the right the right hand comes up in a right ward-off across the body and the left comes across the body at waist level. When your weight is on the right leg and your hands have followed around to hold a ball on the right with the right hand uppermost, then you step out with the left foot and repeat the whole process. In all you step out with the left foot three times.

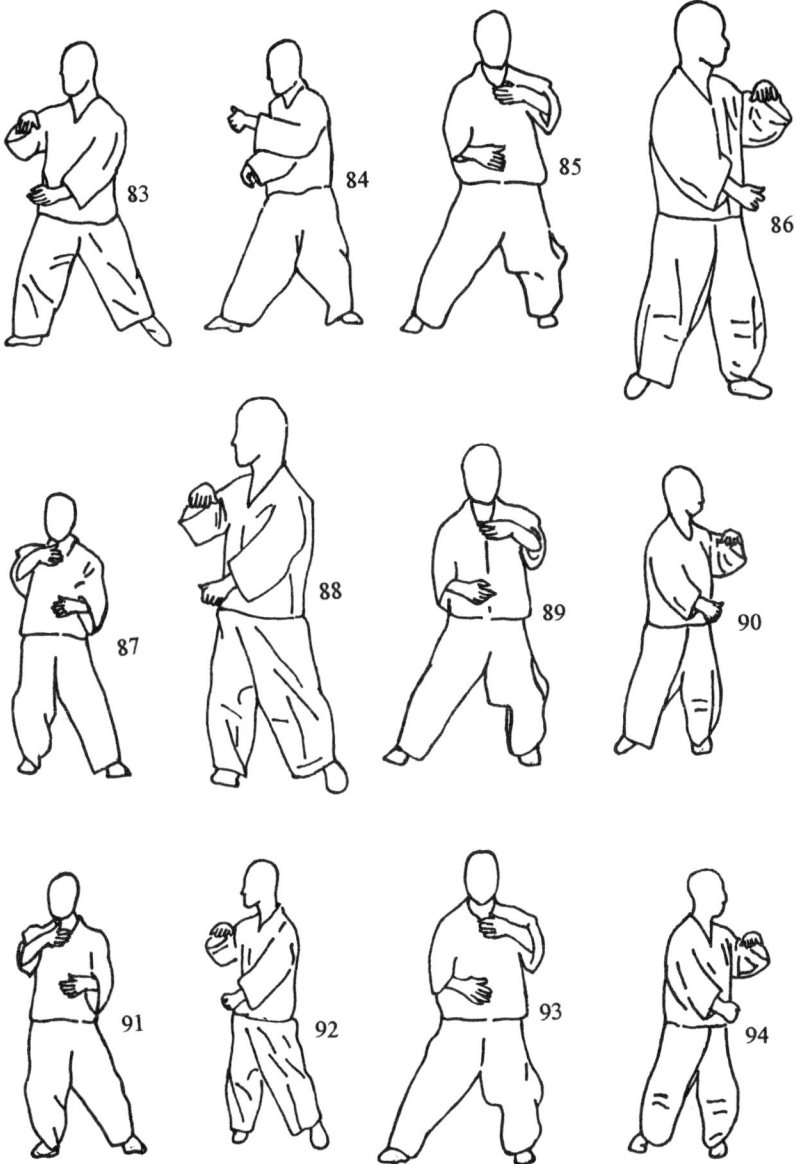

If you want to test whether you are using the waist correctly get a partner to hold lightly but firmly on to either one, or both of your wrists while you perform the movements. You should be able to move your partner around quite easily provided that the waist is being used.

DAN BIAN XIA SHE
Single Whip, low form

This move, popularly called snake creeps down, performs a number of useful functions. In purely physical terms it teaches you how to stretch in a natural and relaxed fashion; while in terms of the tactics of tai chi it shows you how to attack low before you attack high. While you would be unlikely ever to use the principles embodied in this movement in such an extreme fashion, crouching right down close to the ground, you might find yourself evading an attack by ducking low and then pushing up off the ground to counter.

From the last time that you step out to the left when performing cloud hands your right foot takes a step directly to your front. As you do this the right hand comes up in ward-off. The left hand meanwhile comes around at waist level and the right hand turns over so that you are in fact holding a ball. As you do this you will need to turn the waist slightly to the right. From there you turn your waist back to the left, pivoting on the ball of the left foot. The right hand which by now has formed a paw extends out to the right in the same way as it has done when you have performed single whip previously. Then take a slightly longer and wider step forward out into the single whip posture. The reason that you have made your stance larger is to make it easier for you when you sink down.

In order to sink you first turn out the back foot, then you shift your weight back on to the back leg and allow it to bend. As you sink you turn in the front foot slightly so as to keep the front leg slightly bent. As you sink down, the front hand also sinks ending up palm facing to the right with the arm slightly bent. You will find that your hand is level with a point somewhere between your mid-calf and ankle, depending on the length of your arm.

Your waist is facing out to approximately forty-five degrees and so your right hand which is held in a paw is extended to the rear at an angle of forty-five degrees.

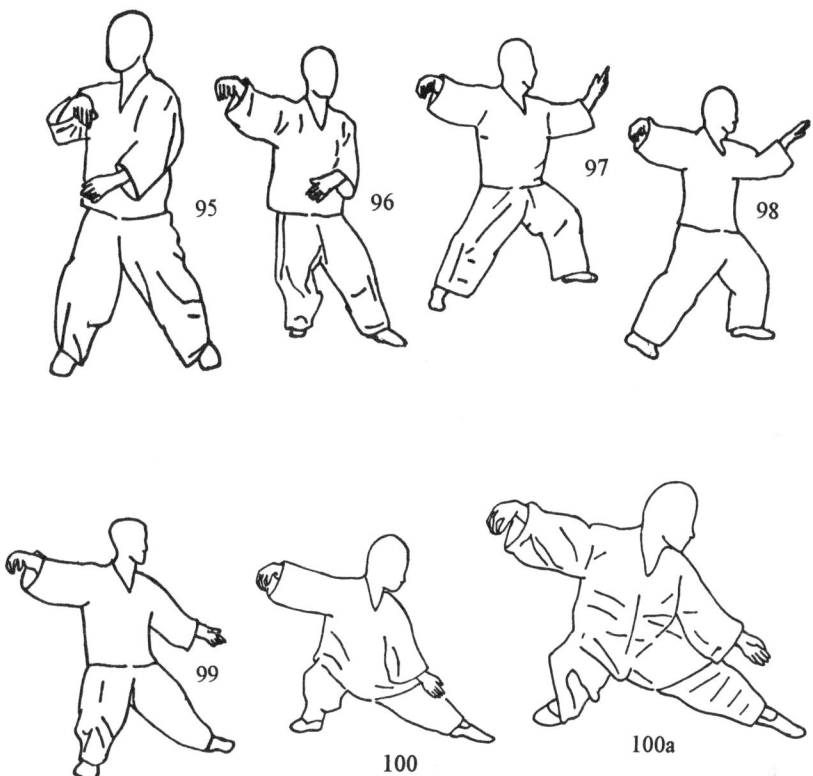

The back thigh must not go lower than being parallel with the ground otherwise you will find that it is difficult to get up as the muscles have gone beyond the angle necessary to give you the required elasticity, rather like a rubber band that has been stretched too far.

This posture will provide you with all the stretching that is needed if you are to be able to apply the full range of tai chi chuan techniques effectively.

JING JI DU LI
Golden Rooster Stands On One Leg

After the previous posture where you have gone low, according to the tai chi principle of the constant interchange of yin and yang, it is only to be expected that you will attack high.

This movement combines a knee strike with a finger attack to the opponent's throat, face or eyes, and in terms of the solo form tests and develops your balance.

From the previous move you turn out the front foot to the left, pivoting on the heel. Then shift your weight forward, adjusting the back heel as necessary. Next, as slowly as you can, bring the back leg forward and up, standing on the left leg.

As your weight is shifted to the front foot, the left hand comes up, palm facing right, fingers pointing upwards and bent at the elbow. At the same time as the back leg steps up, the back hand relaxes down, the paw opens and you move your hand in a semi-circular arc on the vertical plane. So you are executing a rising finger strike, palm facing left. While this hand is rising the other hand drops to rest by the left thigh, palm facing backwards.

Then your right, raised leg steps backwards, to be placed down with the foot at a forty five degree angle so as to form a firm base as you shift your weight on to it. The right hand drops down by the right thigh, palm facing backwards, as the left, knee rises and the left hand comes up to perform the posture on the other side.

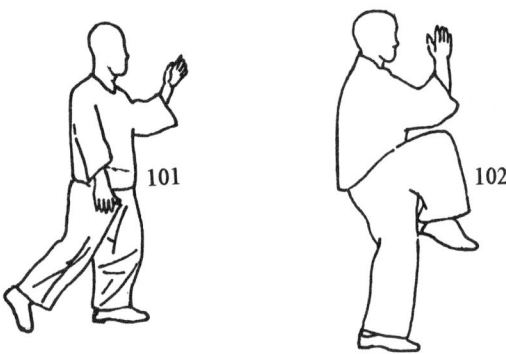
101   102

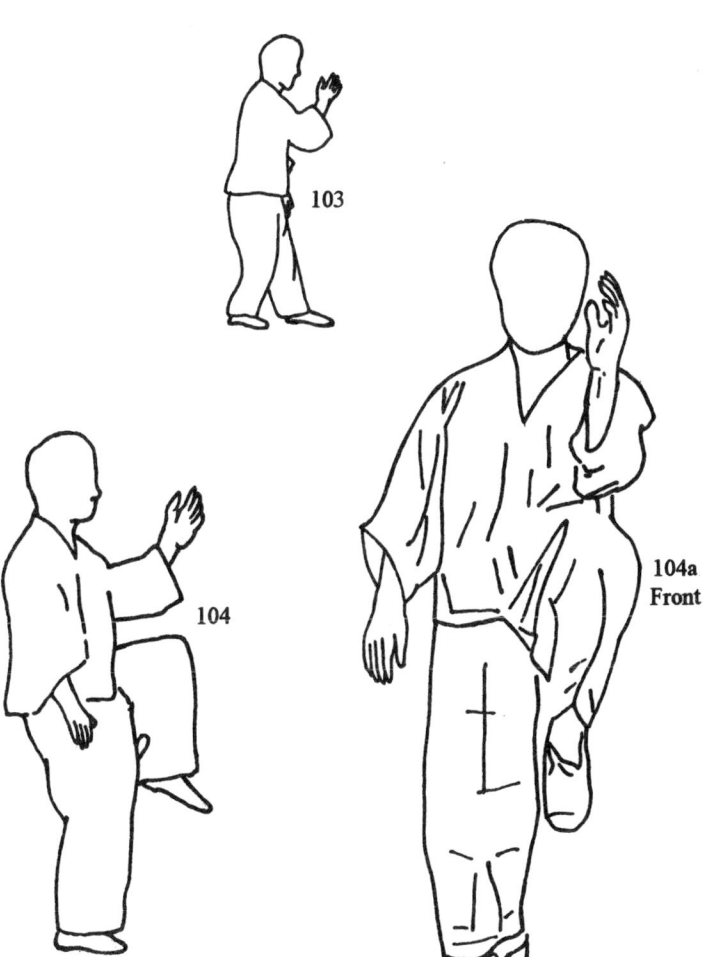

103

104

104a
Front

In practising this move you must take great care that your
movement does not become too sunk or too high. This means that
you must make sure that from the waist down your body sinks with
the supporting knee bent, while the upper half of the body feels as
if it is being pulled up. An added complication in this movement is
that the raised knee should be pushing up to meet the sinking elbow
of the arm on the same side.

ZUO YOU FEN JIAO
Left and Right Toe Kick

From the previous movement the left foot takes a long step back and out to the left and the left hand comes down to hold a ball under the right, with the weight on the right leg.

Then from there shift the weight back on to the left leg and leave the right hand where it is. This appears as if you are moving the right hand out, palm down, but in fact it is the body that is moving away. As the body sits back, turn to the left and execute LU with the right hand; your left hand is already in PENG across the chest.

When you have moved as far as you can to the left, let the left hand drop away and then come over the top in a circle to rest, left wrist on top of right wrist. In order to move the hand your waist has turned slightly to the right.

Then you separate both hands in a semi-circle over and above the head with the hands turning so that they face outwards. As you do this the right leg lifts up, bent at the knee so that you are executing a kick with the toe at about shin height.

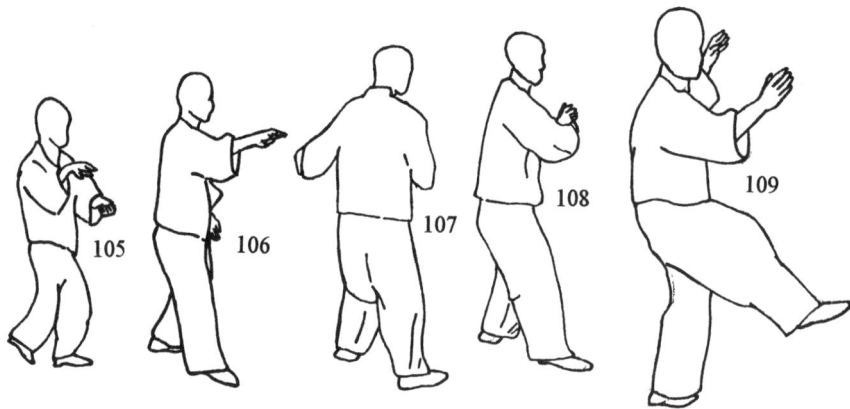

105   106   107   108   109

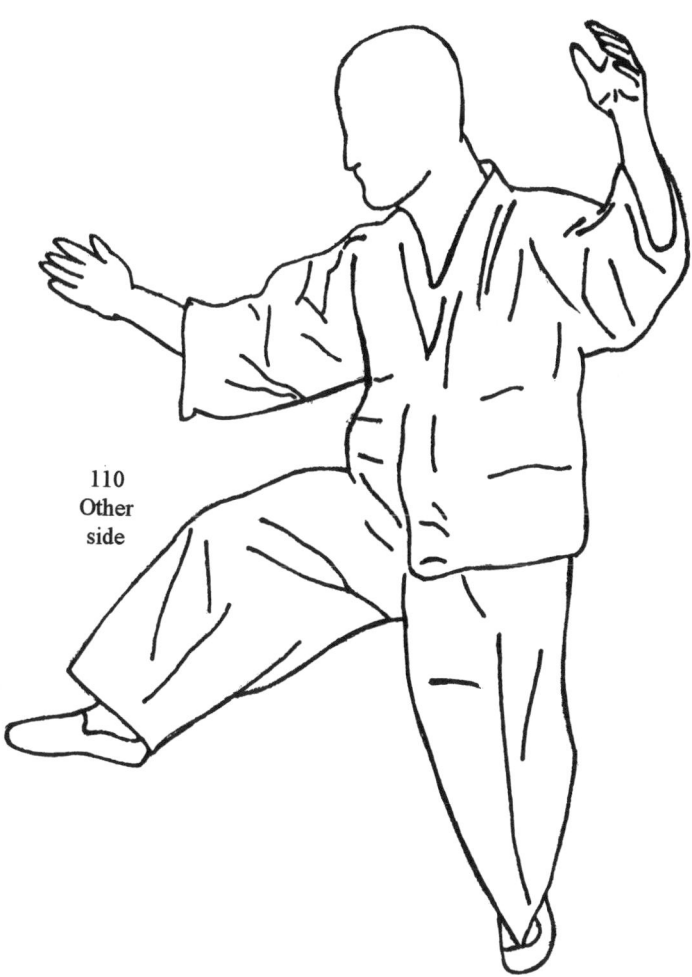

110
Other
side

When you kick your body is turned to the side; a tactically sound move so as to present as small a target as possible. The back hand is slightly higher than the front one so as not to place too much pressure on the front arm/shoulder.

When kicking in tai chi we generally follow the principle of only doing so when you have three legs on the ground! What this means is that the kick is only used when you are close enough to the opponent to grab hold of him.

This movement follows the principle of going high to attack low, or vice-versa. Either you grab the opponent's arm to unbalance or distract him as you kick him in the shin; or the shin kick is a distraction for a high attack.

Next you are going to perform the same technique on the other side. Your right leg which has just kicked, takes a long step back to the right and your hands drop to hold a ball, left hand on top, while the weight stays on the left foot. You then sit back, and turn into Lu, by moving your waist to the right. Next turn your waist to the left to bring the right hand over to rest on top of the left hand. Then kick. This sequence is the same as for the technique on the other side.

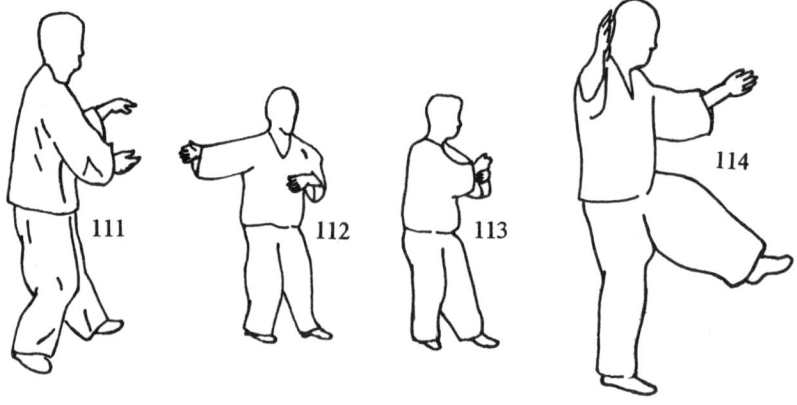

When you perform this move the feeling in your kicking leg is as if you have to pull it up off the ground. If this is too easy, you are using too much muscular tension in the hip area.

When you kick in tai chi the leg must be relaxed so that all the power is transmitted into the target.

ZHUAN SHEN DENG JIAO
Turn Body Heel Kick

In this movement you are practising turning and developing and maintaining balance.

From the Left Toe Kick bring the left foot back and step across and behind your right foot, It is not necessary that the legs should be so close together that they touch. At the same time the right hand drops down and out to the right side, with the hand at waist height, palm facing to your front. The left hand drops across the body so that the hand is placed level with the right hip, palm facing in. You are now prepared to turn.

To make the turn pivot on the right heel and left toe until you are facing your rear. The hands follow the movement of the body round with the left hand coming up across the chest while the right hand comes around to cross it at the wrist, with both palms facing in.

Then raise your left leg from the knee and extend the lower leg but keeping the knee slightly bent. This kick may be executed at any height below the waist.

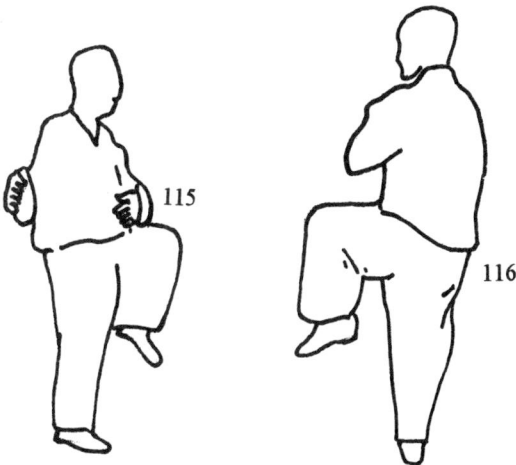

115

116

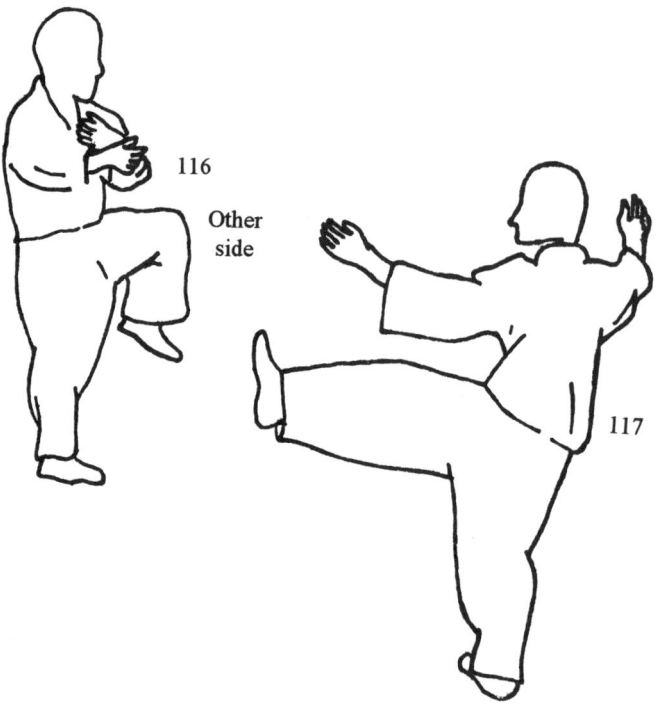

116

Other
side

117

Remember when you kick not only to keep the kicking leg slightly bent but also the supporting one.

In a more advanced version of this move you do not put the left foot down but instead bring it in next to the right foot, keeping the knee raised, and then pivot on the heel of the right foot. Beginners tend to tense their shoulders when turning so it is not a good idea to try this until you have mastered the first method.

Intermediate move from Left Heel Kick into Brush Knee Twist Step.

From the left heel kick, in order to step down into Brush Knee Twist Step you first relax the left leg, from the knee down. At the same time allow the left hand to fold in at the elbow until the left hand rests inside the left knee which remains up. While this is happening the right hand folds over to rest by the right ear as it normally does during Brush Knee Twist Step. Then your left leg steps out, the left hand brushes the knee and the right hand moves forward to complete the posture as the right foot pivots around to the required angle.

You then repeat **Brush Knee Twist** Step on the other side.

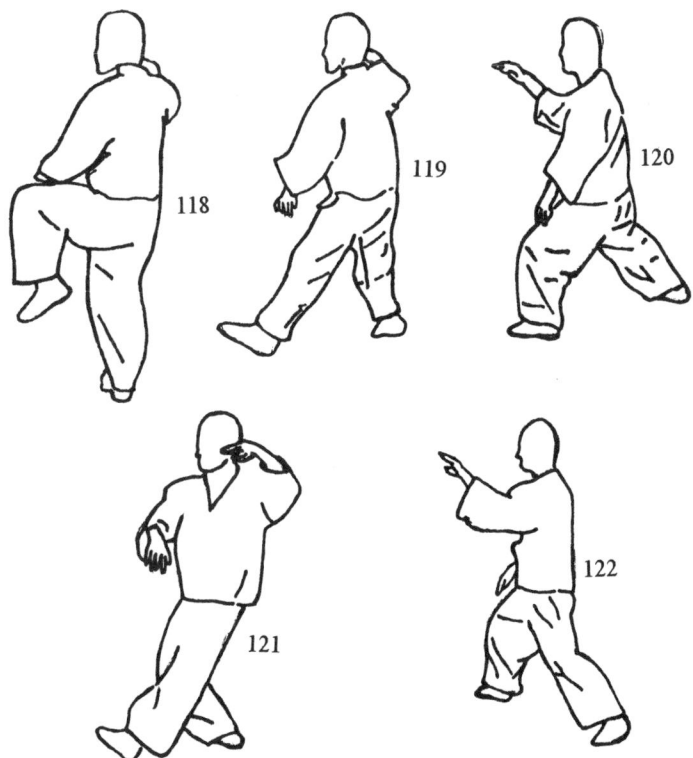

JING BU ZAI CHUI
Step Forward And Plant A Punch

In Step Forward and Plant a Punch as the name suggests you are planting a punch, in this case in the opponent's lower abdomen. The use of the word "plant" suggests a deliberate sinking motion which this posture emphasises.

From the previous move sink back on to the left leg and turn your waist to the right, turning out the right foot as you do so. At the same time the hands drop into the bear position. As you shift your weight on to the right foot the right hand forms into a fist and then your left foot steps out. The left hand brushes the knee and the right hand punches in low. When you get to the end of this movement bend slightly from the waist so that the head inclines forward, thus protecting it.

This move effectively parries a low attack and counters to the opponent's groin. In line with the tactical principles of the art it follows the high attack in Brush Knee Twist Step.

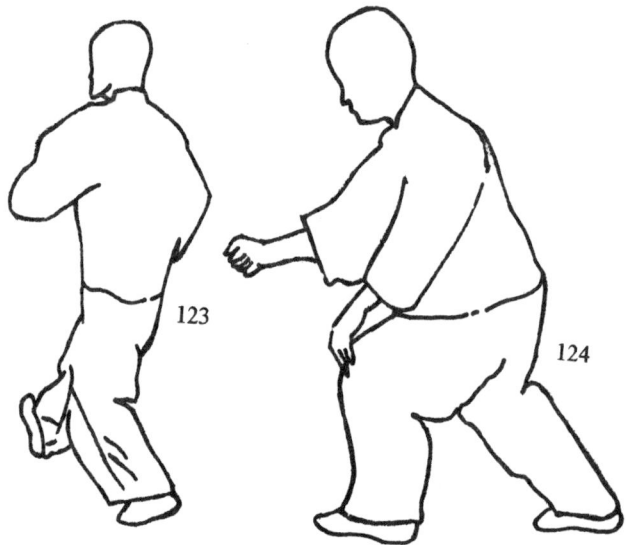

123

124

It is very important in this move that you keep the hips as soft and relaxed as possible. This allows you to drop your weight into the technique.

As with all the other movements where you form a fist, it is made as the weight is shifted onto the appropriate leg; in this way you condition your body to sink when striking thus allowing most effective use of the bodyweight.

JING BU LAN JUE WEI
Step Forward Grasp the Sparrow's Tail

The four moves of PENG, LU, JI and AN are practised exactly as you have done before, but you step forward into them from the previous move. This you do by sitting back on to the right leg and turning the waist to the left. As this happens let your left hand rise slightly and bring your right hand round and underneath it to hold a small ball. Then step through with your right leg and bring both hands up into right ward off. Then execute LU, JI and AN.

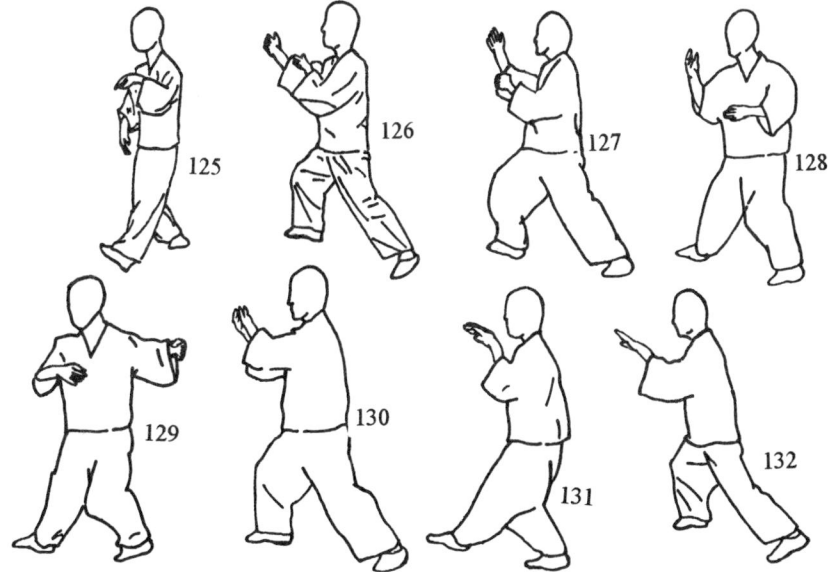

DAN BIAN - Single Whip

Executed as described above.

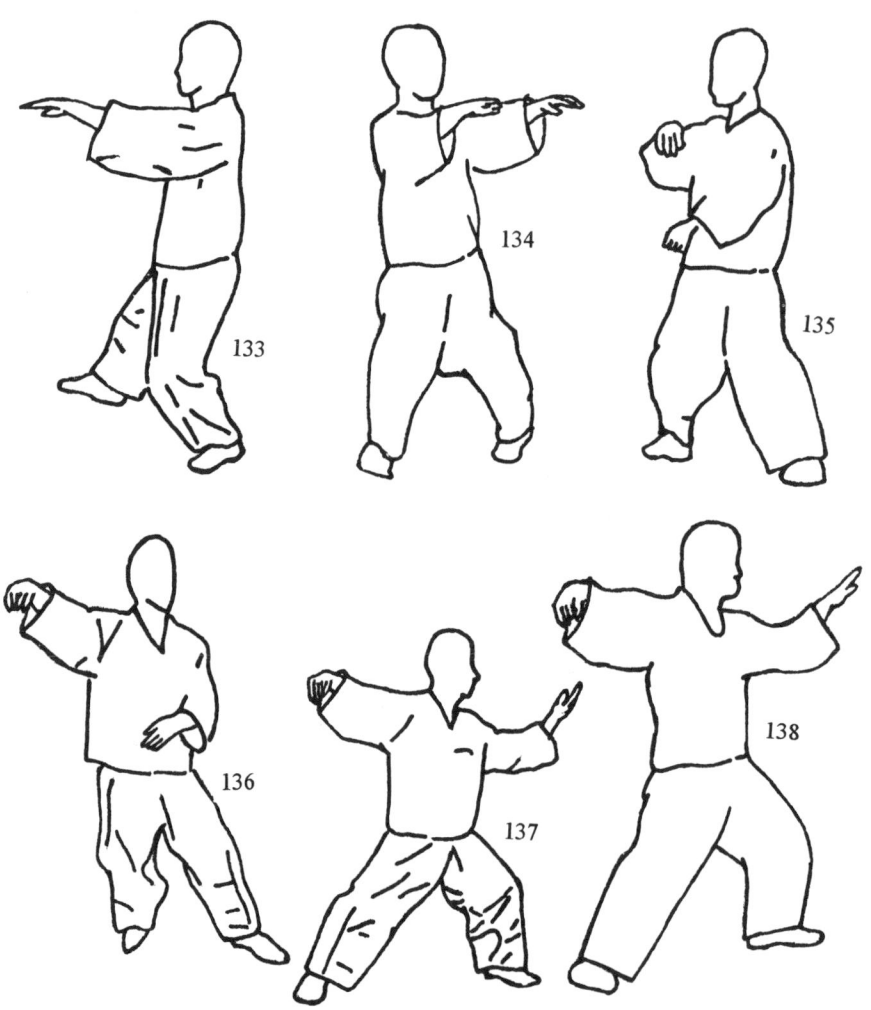

YU NU CHUAN SUO
Fair Lady Plays Shuttles

In this movement you will learn how to shift your weight from one leg to another in the most difficult of circumstances, as you turn and step out to the rear diagonal.

From DAN BIAN you shift your weight on to the back leg allowing the front hand to drop down at the same time. Then turn in the front leg as far as you can. Once your front foot has turned in shift your weight to it and, while this is going on, your back hand opens out from the paw and drops at the elbow, palm down to end up facing the bottom hand, as if holding a ball.

Your right foot then turns out and steps out slightly to your right and you place your weight on it so that you can step through with the left leg to the diagonal. As the weight is shifted to this front leg, the left hand comes up in a semi-circular action with the palm facing into the body as the forearm comes up to the torso and then turns so that the palm is outwards and the forearm above the head as the movement is completed.

The turning of the waist brings up the lower hand, palm facing away, to strike in the direction of any opponent's face. The elbows of both arms stay hanging down.

From here you are going to turn to your left rear diagonal. In order to do so you first sit back on the right leg, dropping both hands so that you are holding a ball with the left hand on top. You turn in your left foot and turn the waist as far as it will go in a clockwise direction, allowing yourself to pivot on the ball or side of the right foot. This right foot then steps out to what is now your right diagonal. As the weight is transferred to it the right hand comes up across the chest as described above, to move up and forward at face level, ending up with the palm facing down.

From the above stance you are going to perform the same movements as you did in the first Fair Lady Plays Shuttles, with your right leg stepping across to the left, after you have sat on to the left leg and dropped your hands into a holding ball position. You must be careful that your right leg does not cross an imaginary line extending directly forward from your left heel, as this would put you in a dangerous position with your legs crossed.

As the weight is shifted on to the right leg, the left leg steps forward and the weight is shifted on to it, the left arm then comes up in a parrying action across the forehead and the right hand comes up to extend forward, palm down, fingers extended out.

In the last of the four Fair Lady Plays Shuttles postures, you move your weight on to the right leg, drop the arms to hold a ball, turn in the front foot and pivot on the ball/side of the right foot and then step out to your right diagonal. You then perform all the movements described above to end up with your right leg forward, right arm above the forehead and left arm out.

In all of the four postures as in many of the other movements of the form the final turning of the waist is accompanied by a turn in of the back foot to an angle of approximately forty-five degrees.

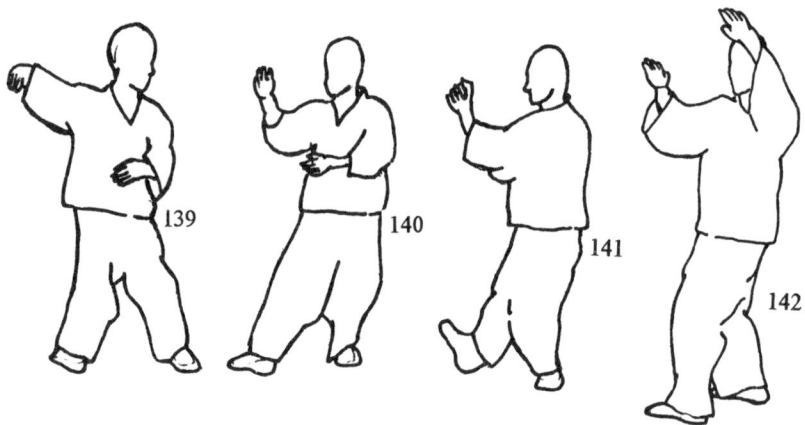

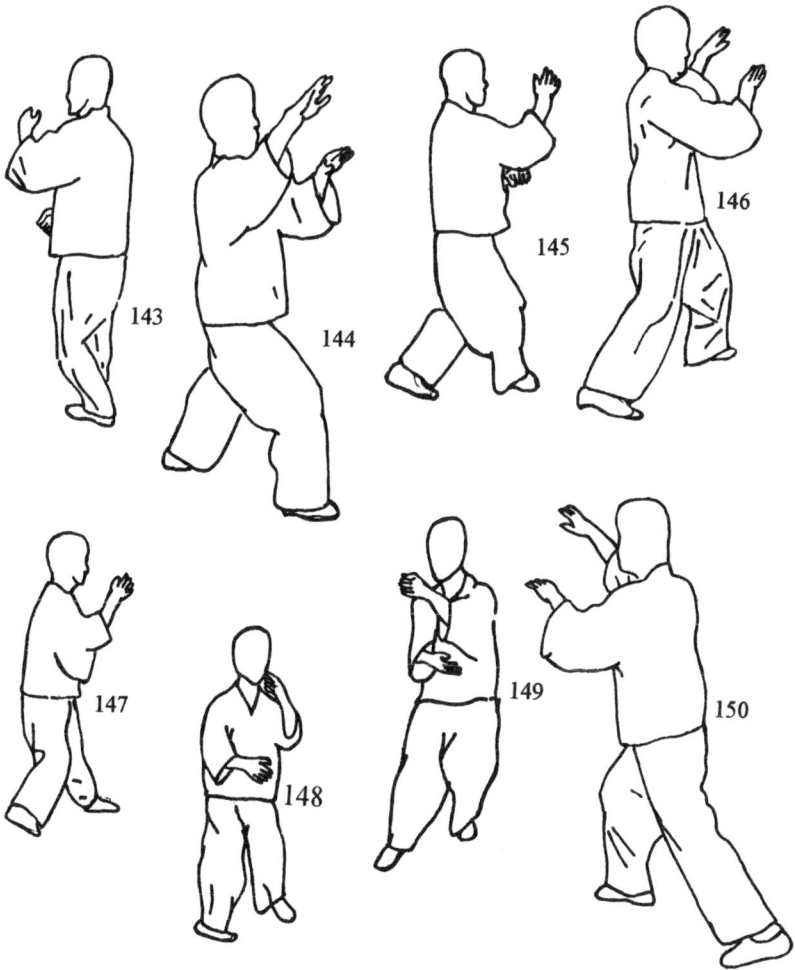

This movement which teaches you how to open the hip joints and turn directly to the rear, the most difficult direction to move in, is also found in the broadsword form.

In order to carry it out successfully you must make sure that when you are turning all of the weight is placed on the supporting foot and the waist is turned as far as possible. This will ensure that the unweighted leg is free to move easily.

Notice how in this movement the waist action is clearly carried on by the shoulder, then the elbow and finally the wrist.

YOU LAN JUE WEI
Right Grasp The Sparrow's Tail

From the previous move you sit back on the left leg and turn in the right foot a little. As you sit back the hands hold a ball, right hand on top. You then turn your waist slightly to the left and step out with your left foot and execute left Ward-Off. You then perform Right Grasp the Sparrow's Tail as you have done previously.

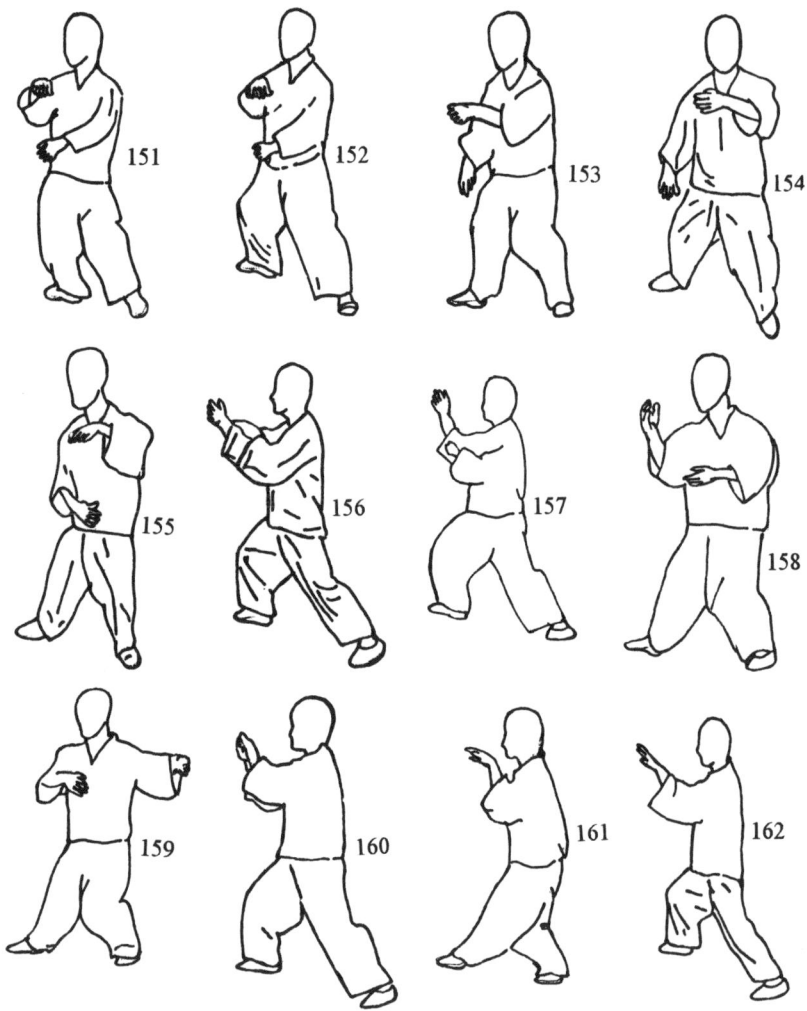

DAN BIAN XIA SHE is then executed as before.

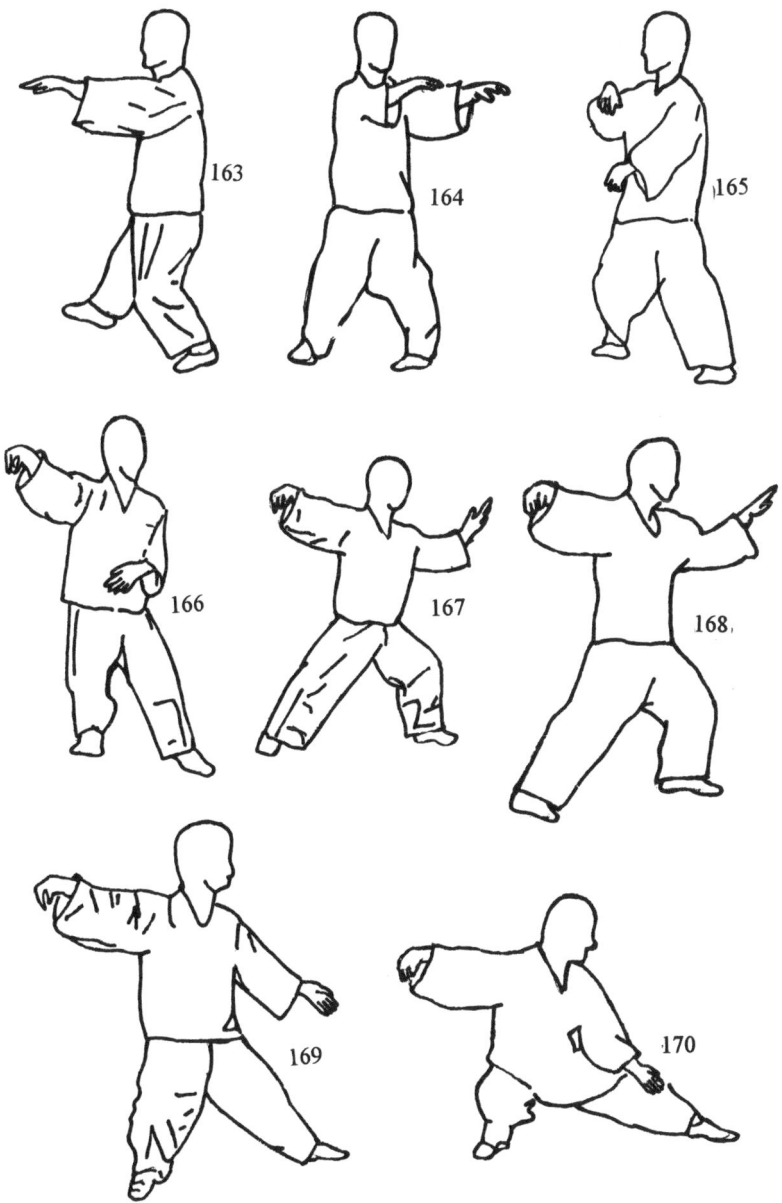

SHANG BU QI XING
Step Up To Seven Stars

You move out of Low Single Whip in the same way that you do when moving into JING JI DU LI, with your left arm coming up. In this move as you bring up your back leg, you do not leave it in the air but still keeping the weight on the left leg, your right leg rests on the ball of the foot. Meanwhile the right hand comes up in a semi-circular vertical arc, forming a fist as it forms a cross in front of your left hand which is also clenched.

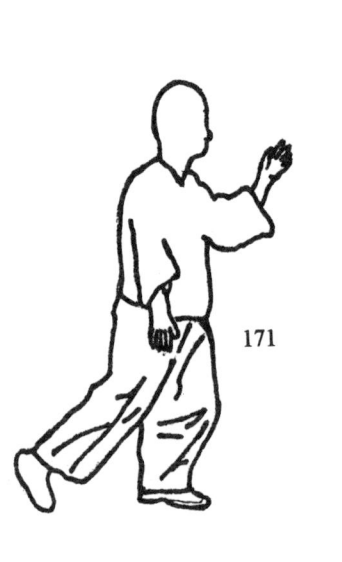

171

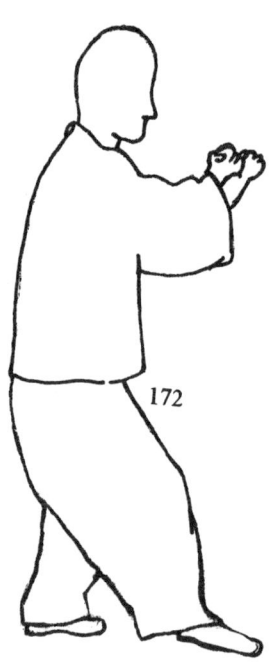

172

This movement might be seen as a double-handed block or a strike with the crossed fists to the throat of an opponent.

The feeling of this movement is of a circular, rising action, with the strain being taken by the front foot while the right foot comes up and steps through.

The principle applied in this movement could also be applied to stepping up to kick.

Be sure to keep your weight relaxed and down on the left leg.

TUI BU KUA HU
Step Back To Ride The Tiger

In Step Back To Ride The Tiger you are emphasising the waist which is truly powerful when you allow it to relax.

The name of this posture encapsulates its purpose for it illustrates the principles you would use to deal with an attack that comes in with great force and great speed. In order to do this you must retreat in order to advance, as the "classics" advise.

Your right leg steps back to the rear as you turn your waist to the right and allow the right hand to drop down to waist level, opening your fingers as you do so. At the same time the left hand drops to the left hip. You then turn the waist to face forward, bringing up the right hand at shoulder height, palm open and facing away from you. With the turning of the waist the left hand moves around the knee to end up in a brush knee position.

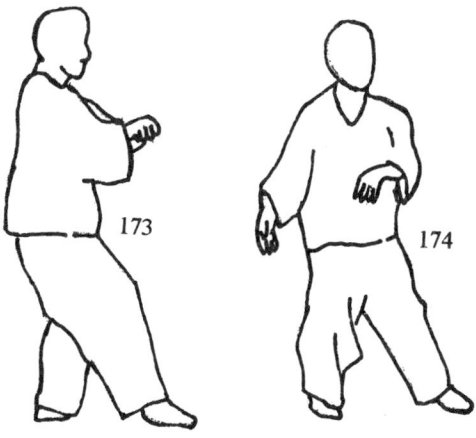

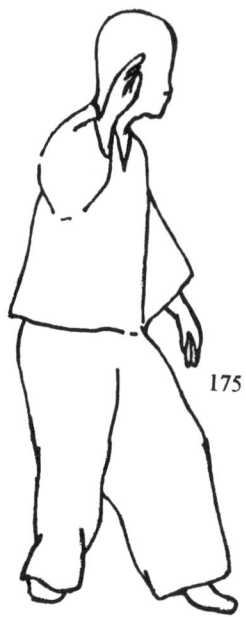

175

This posture somewhat resembles White Crane Spreads its Wings but its intent is different. You have turned your waist and stepped back to avoid your opponent's first onslaught. You then turn back to catch your opponent as he retreats.

ZHUAN SHEN BAI LIAN TUI
Turn Body White Lotus Kick

This movement is as much a test of your balance and posture as an effective fighting technique. Indeed it would in most cases be suicidal to turn your back on an opponent when fighting.

From the previous posture drop both hands. The left hand goes out to your left while the right hand goes across the body. The left palm is facing forward while the right palm faces backwards.

The left leg then circles around clockwise to the rear with the hands coming around and providing the propulsion. As you do this you pivot on the ball of the right foot. You then place your left foot down on the heel directly behind the front foot. Next continue the turn by pivoting on the left heel till you are once again facing the direction you were facing when you executed Step Back to Ride The Tiger. Both your hands then execute a circular motion from left to right and then back, palms down to sweep across the right foot which has moved up and around from left to right in a slow-motion crescent kick. The hands are then brought down by the right side, where they form fists, while the right foot comes down by the left, either lightly resting on the toes or just off the ground .

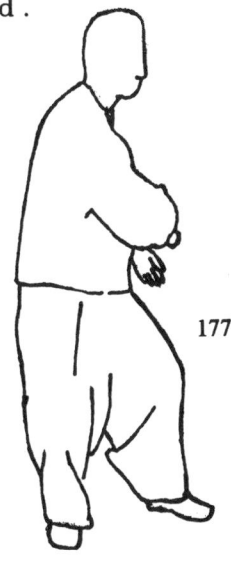

177

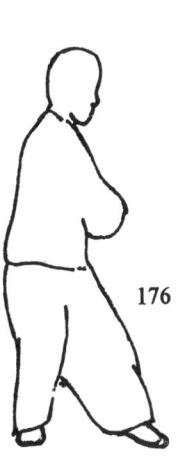

176

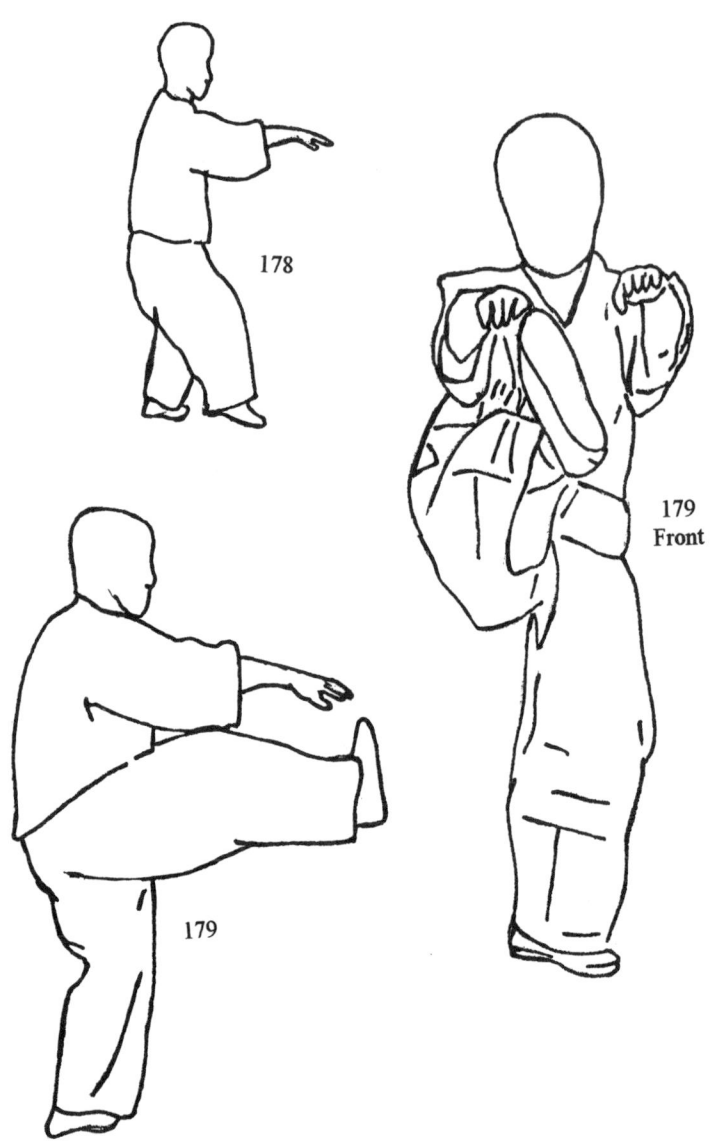

178

179
Front

179

You then move straight into the next move:

WANG GONG SHE HU
Draw A Bow To Shoot The Tiger

Your right leg steps out diagonally to the right into a front stance as your hands draw back slightly to the rear of the right hip and then move in a circle following the action of the waist which turns slightly to the left so as to face the left diagonal. The lower, left hand circles over at stomach height to end up with the fist held vertically facing the same diagonal as the waist. At the same time the upper, right hand circles around slightly behind the right shoulder and then following the movements of the waist to end up at the level of your temple but at least a foot away from it, thumb side down. The appearance and feel of this movement is that of deflecting a low attack and striking the opponent high.

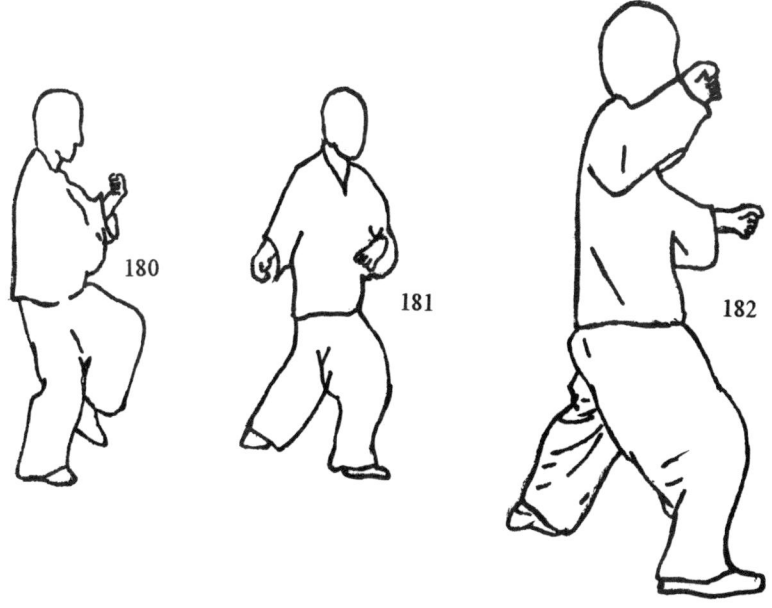

To move into the next posture :

JING BU BAN LAN CHUI
Step Forward, Move, Parry and Punch

Drop your right hand which opens up, palm down, as if it was stroking downwards. The left hand turns palm up and also strokes downwards. As this is happening the back leg steps up half a step and you then turn out the right foot to begin the same moves for this posture that you have carried out before.

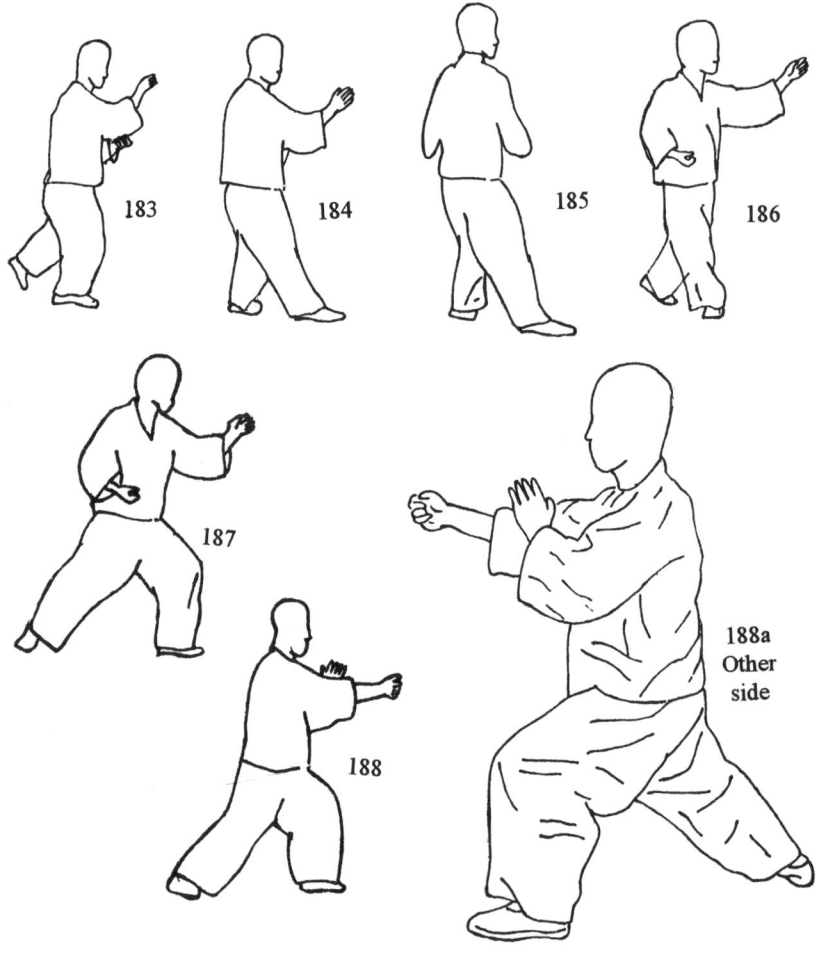

This move is then followed by **RUFENG SIBI**, exactly as you have previously practised it. You then turn, performing exactly the same moves as you did for **SHIZI SHOU** until you have crossed your hands in front of you into **HE TAI CHI** or close the Tai Chi. Both hands drop down to either side, elbows still bent. Then you push the palms down and let the fingers follow them and drop as you straighten your legs. All this time the weight remains on the left leg. You then turn out the right foot to a forty-five degree angle and step the left foot up to it, turning in your palms so that they face your sides as you do so. You have now finished the form.

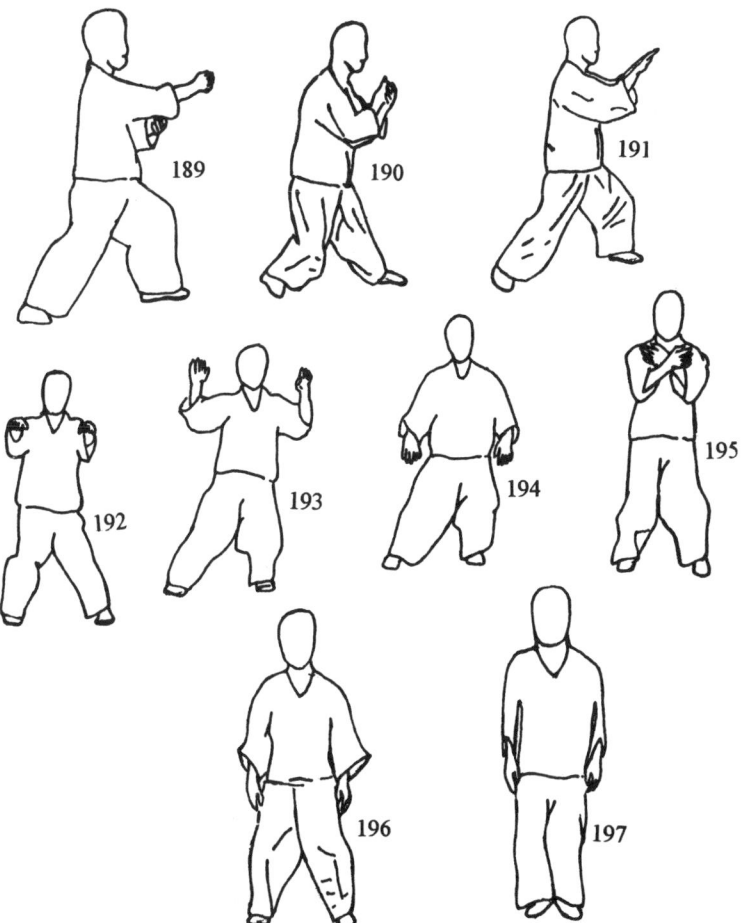

PART TWO

BRANCHES
FROM FORM TO FUNCTION

In the recent history of tai chi chuan there has been much taught that has been confusing, misleading and in some cases just plain wrong. One result of this has been that students of the art spend a disproportionate amount of time concentrating on more or less obscure aspects of the form while failing to place it in its wider context as a part of a system that has a number of aims.

The main aim of those who first created the art was to provide themselves with an efficient martial art. A second subsidiary aim that developed most probably from the way in which the art increased in popularity was the promotion and preservation of good health.

There can be no doubt that tai chi was a martial art first and a health art later, as diligent scrutiny of the historical writings on the art will reveal. But irrespective of whether you accept this statement or not, what is important is that if we accept the martial and the medical as being the two major factors behind the continued growth and development of the art then we have two ways of assessing the effectiveness of our art in application.

This is important because in recent years it has become an increasingly prevalent practice to judge the quality of a person's tai chi by the appearance of the form. This is nonsense for much of what we are seeking to develop is internal. Of course, one can see whether a person is conforming to the general physical principles of the art but it is very difficult to judge whether the person is genuinely relaxed, has the ability to move quickly and in a balanced manner from one posture to another, or has the kind of mental and physical relaxation that may be sustained under pressure.

What must happen next if we are honestly seeking the martial and the medical benefits of the art is that we must remain self-critical and endeavour to create for ourselves realistic opportunities to both practice our skills and test whether they are effective. This does not mean that we should go out and pick a fight at the local 'biker' bar, although I suspect that this would meet with the approval of some of the masters of old, but rather that our training should be specifically designed so that we are constantly compelled to be honest about our progress and abilities.

If I had a five pound note for every time that someone has said to me, while practising either pushing hands or applications, "I could have got you then !", I would be quite wealthy. And certainly sometimes they could have got me, but that is not the point. Through the training I have been compelled to undergo by my teachers, I know that I can take a punch or even several and carry on, I know that pain does not disable me emotionally as it does some people, and I know that even if he does get me it is so only that I can get him back in a big way.

As regards the health aspects of the art we must again take a long and honest look at the state of our own health. Has our practice strengthened the body? Do we find that we are suffering less bouts of cold or flu? Have our bodily functions improved?

It has been my experience and that of other tai chi teachers that I know, that very often those students who seek to learn only the health aspects of the art are the ones who are gaining the least from their practice. Why should this be so?

The answer of course lies in the fact that unless you have a clear understanding of how the martial aspects of the art work you cannot expect to glean the health benefits. This is because the martial art demands that you achieve correct posture in order to harness the full power of the body. This correct posture accords with the way that the body is designed to work and therefore health benefits accrue.

In the light of the fact that we have two measuring sticks for the effective application of the art we shall now go on to consider how the form is applied in martial terms.

STARTING POINTS
APPLYING THE FORM

In this section of the book you will be presented with suggested applications of the principles embodied in the major movements of the form as well as exercises you can practice to develop specific skills.

CHI SHI
Beginning

You can use this movement to practice the basic skill of intercepting the opponent's attack in such a way that you do not unduly interfere with his force. This is done so that you can ascertain the strength and direction of his attack and then use it to your advantage. Of course, all this happens in a split second and the only way that you can acquire the necessary speed is by attaining as relaxed a body and mind as possible. This you do by constant, careful repetition of the form.

Stand opposite a partner and as they extend an arm to point at your face raise both your arms as you would in the form. Of course both your arms will not intercept your partner's arm but one of them will. As this happens you must take care that you do not use excessive speed or force, just let your arm rise up to touch the other person's arm not interfere with it in any direction.

The reason you raise both arms at first is to get you used to using your whole body. Once you feel comfortable performing the move ask your partner to slowly increase the speed of his pointing. When you feel fairly confident stand with your body at a forty-five degree angle to your partner with your right foot just in front of your left. Then as you raise your arms your right arm will automatically be in front and it is this arm that will meet your partner's arm.

It is imperative that you remain both mentally and physically relaxed as you perform this exercise otherwise you will not have the time to make a gentle interception. It is to facilitate your ability to relax that your partner moves slowly and just points rather than punching. Only when you are confident in your ability to remain relaxed should you ask your partner to perform a punching action and then only at a slow speed at first.

Another important lesson taught by this first movement is the power of actions that originate from the waist-hip area. To see this clearly ask your partner to grasp your arms which you have raised to the level of hand position number four of the beginning movements. Now let your arms come down as they do in move number five but make sure that the movement originates from your waist so that your hips sink slightly as the arms come down. At first your partner should provide light resistance which can slowly be increased as you become more used to using your waist.

One further possible self-defence application of these initial movements of the form may be seen in terms of a defence against a two-handed grabbing or choking attack. As the opponent grasps you do not attempt to resist by pulling away. Instead just sink slightly at the knees and then using the ground as a springboard drive your arms up between the opponent's arms in the direction of his face. Even if you do not hit the face the upward movement will break his hold and should startle him enabling you to escape or counter.

PENG, TI SHOU SHANG SHI, YU NU CHUAN SUO
Ward-Off, Lift Hands, Fair Lady Grasps Shuttles

PENG or Ward-Off is one of the eight major manifestations of power in tai chi. As such, elements of it should be present in every tai chi movement.

What we will look at now is some of the specific ways in which it may be used. Again let us imagine an attack with a straight punch. As the punch comes in step forward and raise your hands in the TI SHOU SHANG SHI posture. This should have the effect of stopping the attack. You must step in with your body facing the diagonal so that you present less of a target and this will place one side closer to the opponent and cause one of your arms to come in contact with the opponent's arm. At this point your parrying arm must have PENG energy. In other words it must not collapse under pressure yet it must not be so rigid that you are easily pushed over. You must be able to feel your root so that if needs be you can use your body placement to disrupt the opponent's balance.

From the initial contact with the arm, step your front foot forward into a front stance and raise your parrying arm, this should have the effect of unbalancing the attacker and exposing his flank for your attack which comes in with the other hand. The position you will find yourself in is YU NU CHUAN SUO. In using this posture you must pay careful attention to the way in which the waist is turned once your arm comes into contact with your opponent so that his balance is upset. This will mean that your counter will be twice as effective.

One alternative to simply disrupting the opponent's balance backwards is to use the intercepting arm to grasp his upper arm and pull him forward before executing your counter.

In order to specifically practice the PENG feeling stand in a front stance with your arms either in the same position as ZUO or YOU PENG. If you have a partner available, get them to push using AN against your PENG arm. You should, if you have achieved the correct posture and body alignment, be able to hold off your partner without too much muscular effort. In particular be careful to keep your shoulder relaxed and to use your root. If you are training on your own you can perform the same exercise against a wall or a tree. The latter is better as there is a springy alive feeling about a tree and according to the size of the tree the resistance may be varied.

JING BU BAN LAN CHUI
Step Forward, Move, Parry, Punch

Within this posture are contained three applications of tai chi principles. The right hand that follows the waist around and forms a fist is sometimes known as PI SHEN CHUI and is basically a backfist. This is often best used against the opponent's attacking limb, although it may also be used to good effect against the opponent's face, coming down and across on the diagonal.

There are a number of ways that this might be practised. Obviously this can be done with a partner but if you are compelled to train on your own then you may use a tree branch or other protruding object.

The technique may also be used on a suspended bag or on a sandbag placed on a bench or table at about waist height. This will enable you to practise the necessary relaxation required to make this technique as efficient and effective as possible.

While practising this technique against a partner's attacking limb you must be careful to allow your movements to be relaxed and natural. Mentally you go on automatic pilot, allowing the body to aim and fire. In this way you will be able to hit the target and allow your force to smash into and through the target.

The parrying hand also follows the action of the waist coming around to intercept an attack, assess the nature and direction of the opponent's force and then move in to counter. Alternatively this parrying hand may also be used to destroy the attacking limb with relaxed power that smashes through the target without thought of specific focus.

Again this technique may be practised with a partner. Be careful though for the waist action makes it very powerful and it is probably an idea to have your partner wear some kind of padding on their arm.

The final part of this movement is a punch. A number of lessons may be learnt from the way this works in the form. First of all, as in every other tai chi movement the waist is the initiator and the punch only happens because of the action of the waist. Secondly the target area is the opponent's mid-section or lower abdomen. Since the effectiveness of tai chi does not necessarily rely on you having conditioned fists, when the fist, which is easily broken, is used in attack it is always against a soft or vulnerable part of your opponent. Finally the Chinese character used for fist in tai chi has the connotations of a ball and chain-like action, with the spine as the handle, the arm as the chain and the fist as the ball. What this means is, that there is no cocking or chambering action for the tai chi punch but rather when the opportunity presents itself the fist flies out.

This you may test with the help of a partner. Stand in a relaxed posture facing your partner who is going to attempt to parry or block your attacks. The first few times chamber your fist, either at the hip or shoulder and then punch. Then let your hands drop and the next time you punch allow the arm and fist to simply fly up to hit your partner. This will undoubtedly be successful. That this is so is due to the way that your will is engaged in the punching action. When you deliberately try to hit a specific target you are far less likely to be successful than if you simply let yourself punch and the fist find its own target.

If you have protective equipment, such as chest guards or punching pads you can test your punching power on your partner. Make sure that you get plenty of feedback from the person you are working with. You should be looking for your power firstly to unbalance your partner and secondly to penetrate his body so that he feels some discomfort. Obviously this can only be done a few times and as a test of the power you are developing. If your partner finds the experience too uncomfortable then stop or use more protective equipment.

To practise the whole move get your partner to aim a mid-section punch at you. As it comes, sidestep to the outside and use a backfist action to strike the attacking arm. As you put your outside foot down, use the outside arm to upset your opponent's balance while you punch in with the other hand.

LU, SHOU HUI PIPA
Rollback, Strum the Lute

As described in the section on the form we can examine LU in terms of two major variations, short and long.

The practice of short LU takes the form of a parry, but you must take care that you also use PENG energy so that you can unbalance your opponent.

Practising against a straight punch you can use this technique either from the inside or from the outside. In both cases, however, you must take care to use the appropriate footwork.

In all these examples we will imagine that you are standing in a right natural stance. This stance with the right foot slightly in front of the other, with the front foot pointing forward and the back foot at forty-five degrees, has a number of advantages. Firstly it enables you to shift your weight easily from one leg to the other thus facilitating speedy movement. In addition with the hands hanging loosely and naturally at your sides you do not present a threatening appearance to any potential adversary, thus your martial arts ability will be augmented by the surprise factor.

In the case of use of LU from the outside, your left foot steps diagonally forward, placing you out of the way of the opponent's strike and enabling you to place your left arm in a LU position covering the opponent's elbow. This leaves you free to step in with the right foot and counter with either hand.

When using LU to the inside, step your left foot behind the right and to the right diagonal and then immediately step in with the right foot. In using footwork to both left and right, when you step in you do so to the diagonal, "through" the opponent's stance in the direction in which it is weakest.

By moving your left foot behind, the upperbody is moved out of the way of the attack. At the same time your right hand performs a short Lu covering action. Then as you step in, this front arm which is closest to the opponent, may be used to attack.

The same footwork may be used with long LU, as it may with almost any tai chi technique, but in considering how to apply LU and turn it into an unbalancing movement or a lock we practise it with a step back.

Now, according to tai chi principles we go back to move forward, so in this case we shall work with an extremely strong and fast attack. As the opponent steps in, step sharply back with the right foot, at the same time intercepting the attacking limb with both hands, one on the wrist and one on the elbow. Once you have grasped the opponent turn your waist to the right and pull down to a forty-five degree angle. Do not worry if the opponent tries or is able to resist, for when he attempts to pull back, follow him and use one or other of the hands to strike him in the face. Immediately you must move forward so as to abide by tai chi tactical principles.

This LU may be converted into Strum the Lute. This is done by straightening the opponent's arm as you roll it back and then grasping the opponent's elbow with the forward hand. Then roll anti-clockwise your hand which is holding the attacker's wrist so that the palm faces down, while the other hand rolls around anti-clockwise, so that it ends up under the opponent's elbow, pushing up to put pressure on the elbow joint. At the same time you step forward pushing both arms up so that the opponent's straightened arm is pushed up into the shoulder joint.

Another classical application of LU as an armbreaking technique, is one which places emphasis on footwork, and although it might not be terribly practical it does serve as a useful training method.

Get your partner to step in with either leg and to punch with the same side. If the attacker steps in with the left foot, punching with the left hand, your left foot steps around his front leg as your left hand uses PENG to intercept his attacking arm. Your right foot then follows round and your right arm executes LU against the elbow joint. Your right foot should be placed into the opponent's stance, that is between his legs. This will help to unbalance him.

XIE FEI SHI , DAN BIAN
Diagonal Flying, Single Whip

Diagonal Flying embodies the principles both of CAI and LIE. Cai, which is normally translated as pluck is an action whereby you take an incoming attack and, grasping the limb, jerk your opponent off balance. LIE, translated as splitting, consists of using an attacking force in one direction while also applying force in another direction at the same time.

Therefore in Diagonal Flying we see the lower hand pulling the opponent's attacking limb down while the other hand strikes up to the attacker's face or throat.

To practice this move with a partner, if he is punching with his right fist use your left arm to intercept in PENG. This left hand then turns anti-clockwise over the top of the attacking arm and pulls it down. As the opponent is jerked off-balance you step in with the right leg and strike up along the opponent's arm with your right hand. Your strike is with the thumb side of the hand, palm facing upward.

In order to practice the skill of CAI, stand opposite your partner with both of you standing in a natural shoulder-width apart stance. Both of you should hold your right arms up in PENG, touching at the wrist. Then you take it in turns to execute CAI. You must try and do this without telegraphing your intentions. In order to do this your touch must be as light as possible and when you pull down use only one or two fingers and the thumb. This will stop you from grasping too tightly and so being unable to swiftly release your hand should you need to do so.

The next step is to practice CAI in the context of double hand pushing hands. Again the watchword must be sensitivity as you are trying to catch the opponent by surprise and take them off-balance. This is so that your counterattack is as effective as possible.

DAN BIAN may also be used instead of the side of hand strike described above so that after you have intercepted the opponent's punch and pulled it down, as you step in your right hand strikes upwards in an uppercut action, impacting with the back of the wrist to the jaw. This technique also applies the principle of LIE, as one hand is being taken down while the other strikes up.

LOU XI AO BU
Brush Knee Twist Step

In applying this technique your parrying hand executes an initially horizontal interception of the attacker's limb down and out to the side thus opening him up for the counter with the other. The striking hand goes in to the target area, fingers first then as the degree of resistance is assessed the palm strikes in. This ensures that the opponent is caught off-balance.

Of course you may not have time to take the opponent's striking arm in the full circular action, in which case you simply jam it in against his chest using PENG energy to disrupt the attacker's balance and set him up for the palm strike.

Another way that this technique may be used is against a kicking attack. First you sidestep, either to the left or right. Then your lower hand is used as a guard to ensure that the kick cannot change direction while the other hand counters. It might be that you are lucky enough to grab the kicking leg with the lower hand, in which case you would unbalance the opponent before striking him. It must be stressed that to use your arm to actually block a kicking attack is extremely dangerous due to the weakness of the arm in comparison to the leg.

TAI CHI KICKING TECHNIQUE

JING JI DU LI, FEN JIAO, DENG JIAO, BAI LIAN TUI & DAN BIAN XIA SHI
Golden Cock Stands On One Leg, Toe Kick, Heel Kick, White Lotus Kick, Low Single Whip

Kicks in tai chi are almost always used in conjunction with upper body attacks, following the principle of going low to attack high and vice-versa. Remember the tai chi saying that you only kick the opponent when you have three legs on the ground, that is you are always close enough to grab the opponent and use his two legs as well as your own for balance.

FEN JIAO, or toe kick is most often used against the opponent's shin as you step in, closing the gap, moving in to strike the head or upper body. In this way your opponent's mind is on the pain in the shin as you hit him in the face.

When practising this technique take care that you do not telegraph with your shoulders. Practice against a partner who steps in with a punch. Intercept the punch with TI SHOU SHANG SHI and then kick with your front leg.

To practice accuracy in this technique get a partner to hold a length of dowelling or a broomstick on which you have made a mark at shin height. Your partner moves around holding the stick out in front of him while you practice your shin kicks on it.

DENG JIAO, the heel kick is used when you are closer in to the opponent and works particularly well when you have seized one of the attacker's arms and are pulling him in towards you. Your heel may then be jammed in to his groin, hip or lower abdomen. The foot may be turned either in or out slightly, depending on your position relative to the attacker. This is an extremely powerful technique and may be practised against trees or a heavy bag so that you get the feeling of impact.

JING JI DU LI is a knee strike, that in the form follows the low form single whip. This is important in so far as it illustrates the principle of going from low to high. While in the form DAN BIAN XIA SHI is done in an exaggeratedly low fashion, in a fight it would be suicidal to execute such a move. Instead as the opponent strikes you might seize his arm and pull it downwards, sinking at the knees. This is done precisely in the hope that he will pull away in an upwards direction so that you may step in and use your knee. At the same time your front hand may be used to strike his throat or face. The same hand may also be used to grasp him around the neck and pull him on to your knee technique.

The inside crescent kick that is poetically called BAI LIAN TUI, or sweep the lotus kick is almost always aimed at the opponent's kidney area, as both the hands grasp the opponent's arm. As in all of the tai chi kicks, because you are operating at close range the knee must be kept bent. In fact this greatly contributes to the springy penetrating power of these techniques.

YUN SHOU
Cloud Hands

As mentioned in the section on form, Cloud Hands particularly stresses the importance of waist action. In application it might be applied as a combination of LIE and CAI, with the top hand intercepting an attack, grasping the attacking limb and pulling the attacker off-balance while the other hand executes a backfist to the body. The waist is used first to jerk the opponent forwards and then is turned to give impetus to the strike.

Another possible application of this move involves grabbing the opponent's arm with one hand while the other goes on the far side of the opponent's arm to execute a lock and ultimately an arm break. This will only work if your left hand is used to grasp the opponent's right hand from the inside, or your right hand grasps the opponent's left hand from the inside.

To practice the use of the waist in Cloud Hands let your partner grasp one or both of your hands while you run through the move as practised in the form. If you use your waist correctly you will find that you can quite easily control them, jerking them around your body which remains quite stable.

BAI HE LIANG CHI
White Crane Spreads Its Wings

White Crane Spreads it Wings is an expansive movement which is usually classically explained in terms of a simultaneous low and high parry. This however would only seem to be required in response to an extremely unorthodox attack.

The principles expressed in this movement can also be used as a defence against a double-handed grab. As your partner takes hold of you sink your weight on to your back leg and turn your waist slightly in that direction. As you do so keep your arms relaxed by your sides but take care to maintain a small space under the armpits. This gives you room to move and will aid you in using the power of your whole body. Having wound up the spring energy in your back leg by sinking on to it, a movement you have practised many times in the form, you release it as you turn your waist back to the front and one arm raises up and to one side while the other goes down to the other side. This should be sufficient to break the opponent's hold after which you can allow your upraised hand to strike down on the attacker.

BAO HU GUI SHAN
Embrace Tiger Return To Mountain

This movement may best be seen as a response to an unexpected attack from the rear. As you step round one hand guards low and the other high.

Another possible use of this technique is suggested in SAN SHOU where it takes the form of a parry downward followed by a punch. This would suggest that the movement found in the solo form is somewhat abbreviated and what we perform as a sitting back action together with a lifting of the back hand actually symbolises a strike.

JING BU ZAI CHUI
Step Forward and Plant a Punch

In this technique you are striking low to the opponent's groin or lower abdomen. At the same time you parry a strike using a Brush Knee motion. What is important to note in this technique is that you incline your head. This serves two purposes : firstly it protects your own face, ensuring that you are not butted or struck ; secondly it may also be used as a butting attack.

Remember that to accord with tai chi principles you should practice this low technique in combination with attacks to higher or lower target areas.

Another point that must be borne in mind is that the force comes from the sinking of the hips and the turning of the waist.

DAO NIAN HOU
Step Back Repulse Monkey

As noted in the section on form, this movement enables you to maintain your balance while moving backwards. It also enables you to counterattack at will, embodying the principle of retreating to advance.

To gain confidence with this way of moving get your partner to hold your hands applying light resistance as you move through DAN NIAN HOU. You will soon feel that the pulling down action of one hand brings your opponent accelerating onto the other. Indeed this could be one possible application of the move, as a defence against a single wrist grab. Remember when you practise this that it is the sinking and turning of your waist that does the work.

Very similar to the previous application is that of the lower hand parrying an attack as you step back, while the other hand strikes in. This may be taken one step further with the addition of a forward step as you strike so that you step back to step forward.

A third and extremely useful way of practising this technique is as a defence against grappling. Your partner should grab you and attempt to pull you in to their body, while you take one step back, but allow your forward hand (the same side as the forward leg) to stay in contact with their body. The step back should serve to free one side which can then be used to counter. The range should be perfect as it is measured out by the hand that remains in contact throughout the engagement.

To gain the most from this technique you must also practise taking several steps back in the face of a heavy onslaught before delivering your counter. At first to check that you are stepping back correctly get your partner to push against you as you move back so that you are forced to use your back foot to root.

ZHOU DI KAN CHUI
Fist Under Elbow

If you look at Fist Under Elbow exactly as it is executed in the solo form then it is difficult to see how it can be applied. The principle, however, is that one hand is used to intercept an attack while the other hand uses the parrying hand as an aiming point. Simply put you aim to hit your own hand, but of course the opponent's limb or body is placed in the way. This ensures that you can be accurate.

To practise this with a partner you may parry with your right hand, aiming to intercept the strike at the elbow, your other hand is then used to strike the attacker's elbow.

SHANG BU CHI XING , TUI BU GUA HU
Step up to Seven Stars, Step Back to Ride a Tiger

The first move follows the low form Single Whip, following the principle of attacking low to attack high. You might practice this move as a cross block against a devastating attack, or else as an attack to the opponent's throat using the point where the hands cross as the striking weapon.

This move, as applied as a block, may then be turned into a grab with the forward hand which is then pulled back and down, thus unbalancing the opponent. At the same time you step back and, covering the opponent's arm with your front hand, release the grip of the other hand and strike the attacker in the face.

The movement you have just performed is TUI BU GUA HU, Step Back to Ride a Tiger. Important things to pay attention to in this move are the way the waist is used to turn the attacker's force and then counter.

RUFENG SIBI
Apparent Close Up

This movement teaches you how to use neutralising and folding to turn an opponent's attack into an opening for your own counter.

Your partner attacks with a straight punch which you intercept. You then use your other hand to slip under your own arm and to take control of the attacker's limb. Your other hand is then freed to counter. In the process you can step in, taking you closer to your opponent so that there is more power in your counter.

There are an infinite number of variations in terms of the counters you can apply. You might like to try a slap to the side of the face, a punch to the ribs or a ridgehand technique to the neck.

You will also find this technique extensively practised in pushing hands as it gives you the ability to "close down" the opponent, making them vulnerable to your push.

SHI ZI SHOU
Cross Hands

Cross Hands is an opening up move and may be used to expose an attacker's unprotected areas to your counters. As with RUFENG SIBI this is most clearly seen in pushing hands.

To practice this move for self-defence your partner should employ a two-handed grip on the chest or a front strangle. You should bring up your hands, crossing them under the attacker's grip. As you do this, sink one hip and turn slightly to the same side. This will have the effect of breaking the opponent's balance so that you can continue the rising, opening action of the hands, breaking his grip and exposing the chest region to counterattack.

JI
Press

Press involves adding one force to another and as such it can best be seen as an interception followed by a strike to the same area. For example you might step outside a punch, parrying it with the forward arm, after which your other arm would come in to strike crushing the opponent's attacking arm against his body, throwing him off balance as you counter.

AN
Push

While we practise pushing in pushing hands, it is not used as an end in itself in application. Instead it is normally employed to take the opponent off balance so as to make your follow-up techniques more effective. In this light you can go through many of the other movements from the form and look at the way in which they employ pushing actions to set up the main technique. In order to practise AN you might consider JING BU BAN LAN CHUI, RUFENG SIBI, LOU XI AO BU and many others.

PART THREE

GAINING FROM THE EXPERIENCE OF THE PAST
THE CLASSICS

All of the often very colourful imagery used in the teaching of tai chi has a practical application to your own practice of the solo form. The only limit is your own creative imagination.

What follows is an examination of some of the advice given in the classics, that collection of the wisdom and advice of several generations of tai chi practitioners. This is not meant to be the final word but rather to stimulate you to undertake your own research.

As this book is only concerned with the solo form I have restricted my examination to its relevance to that area of practice although all of this advice may be related to any aspect of the tai chi curriculum.

Sink the qi to the dantian

Qi as a concept has many different meanings in Chinese and it is hard to isolate any particular one with reference to tai chi. Here, however, we are dealing with what might best be described as a psycho-physical force, life energy if you like. This energy moves constantly around the body; its movement, however, may be consciously stimulated by the mind. Therefore in heeding this piece of advice we simply have to "think" of the dantian.

The dantian point, also sometimes referred to as the field of qi, is about three finger widths below the navel, and slightly nearer to the front of the body than the rear. In Chinese thought it is an energy centre, but more importantly to tai chi practitioners it also corresponds to the body's centre of gravity.

Bearing this in mind we then find that what we are being advised to do is to think of our centre of gravity; to be aware of our centre of gravity. This is obviously very important advice for anyone practising a system of unarmed combat, where the maintenance of balance is essential.

What we must also bear in mind is the word "sink" as it is also of great importance to the tai chi practitioner. All of our movements must have that sunken feeling. The practical effects of this are that our centre of gravity is lowered and all of the muscles of the upper body are relaxed so that the weight is all resting on the legs.

What does all this mean in terms of form practice?

Once you have come to grips with learning the movements you must then try to "place your mind in the dantian," that is to think of the centre of gravity in every movement you do. This will make you feel much more solid and rooted and will go a long way to ensure that you move from the waist, making the most efficient use of the large, powerful muscle groups in the lower abdomen.

In addition such practice will help you to hone your ability to focus the mind, concentrating on one point, while also moving the body through the form. This ability to remain mentally and physically centred will come in very handy when you move on to pushing hands and fighting training.

Move like a tiger, gaze like a hawk.

In applying this piece of advice to our form practice we have to be selective in choosing which attributes of these two animals we wish to emulate.

In the case of the tiger we are concerned with the relaxed, padding movements which contain the potential for swift and terrible action should it be required. If you study the way a tiger moves you will notice how once its leg touches the ground the whole of the bodyweight follows, yet without jarring and in a relaxedly-controlled manner.

When practising the form we should move like a tiger in slow-motion, full of powerful grace and in command of our environment. Our every movement should also contain the kind of relaxed awareness that may instantly be translated into active response should danger threaten.

Gazing like a hawk involves making full use of the eyes, including the peripheral vision so that as we do form we are aware of all that goes on around us, but are not fixated on any one object. Like the controlled awareness in movement of the tiger, the gaze of the hawk is not startled because it is aware of all that is going on around.

Generally speaking, in the form the eyes follow the movement of the front hand but they do not stare fixedly for this would preclude the use of peripheral vision. This type of vision is most obviously used in Step Back Repulse Monkey where the head follows the body but the eyes must be able to see out of their corners the fingers of both hands.

Raise the 'Spirit of Vitality' to the Top of the Head

The "spirit of vitality" is better expressed as awareness or alertness and therefore what is meant by this is the ability to remain alert.

There are a number of reasons for such advice being necessary for the tai chi practitioner. Firstly there is a tendency when doing the form, because of the need to sink and relax, for the body to become dull and the performer to feel sleepy. By reminding you to keep your alertness at the top of the head you counter this tendency.

The second point is that this has the effect of holding the head as if suspended from above; so that from the waist down there is a feeling of sinking. This internal dynamic tension is what prevents tai chi from being just sluggish movement.

In terms of training the student for fighting this piece of advice is of vital importance as it keeps you alert and best able to respond to the opponent's slightest move.

The duality of the tai chi is also responsible for this piece of advice as where there is a sinking of the body there must be a raising of the mind.

Power is rooted in the feet, released through the legs, controlled by the waist and expressed in the fingers.

While, at first reading, this passage might seem only of direct relevance to the practice of pushing hands or fighting, it is, in fact, of fundamental importance to all areas of tai chi study. It is from the form that you learn the movement principles upon which every other aspect of tai chi is based therefore this passage must be applied to every movement.

Tai chi's power is borrowed from the earth, indeed there is a saying much loved by tai chi practitioners that you must "borrow the strength of the earth and the qi of the heavens". What this borrowing from the earth means in practical terms is that you align the body in such a way that you sink down into the ground like a spring being compressed. The spring is actually your sinews which store up potential energy which can then be released as the situation requires.

In terms of pushing this would mean that when someone pushes you your body must relax so that his force is directed into the ground, then when he relaxes the pressure, the energy will be released pushing him away.

Of course when practising the form no one is pushing us but we are working against a force, that is the force of gravity. So throughout the solo form we are training to feel the power rooted in the feet by letting ourselves relax down and aligning the body so that force is transmitted down from one joint to the next until it reaches the ground.

As you practise the form you will notice that you are constantly storing up power in one leg then releasing it, and it is this process which the passage refers to.

Releasing this power through the legs means that the force comes up from the ground and is not impeded by incorrect stance or tension in the legs. That it is controlled by the waist means that the large muscles of the abdomen, the centre of gravity and the heaviest part of the body direct the force in whichever direction it needs to go.

Expressing power through the fingers points more to what the hands and arms do not do. They are merely a conduit for the "expression" of power that has come up from the ground. So it is that you may visualise the body as a large hose. The source of the water is the ground; the feet are the connection; the direction of the flow is determined by the waist and the fingers serve as the nozzle.

Following this analogy, when doing the form you must take great care to ensure that the hose is never blocked - that the body is aligned in accordance with natural physiological principles and classical advice. As far as the fingers are concerned this means that the "fair lady's hand" must be retained, as bent or unduly straightened fingers will prevent a free flow.

The body stops but the mind does not

Beginners are often surprised that the learning process involves moving from one static position to the next with little of the graceful, flowing that they had hitherto associated with the art. Indeed it is not until you have reached a degree of competence in achieving and holding the correct postures that you will be encouraged to become more flowing.

Even at a high level, however, the master practitioner will be observed to hold each posture momentarily before going on to the next. The reason for this is the same as for the beginner; to ensure that the posture is correct and conforms to all the requirements of the art.

But, as this piece of advice suggests the mind does not stop or go into neutral. Instead it is already moving on to the next posture and initiating the subtle movements that will lead into it.

Throughout the form the mind is aware yet seeking stillness in movement, movement in stillness. Therefore you must endeavour to ensure that although your body might appear to have stopped the mind continues both in awareness and in preparation for the next movement.

Where there is up there is down, where there is forward there is backward, where there is left there is right.

This is obviously embodied in every movement of the form and is what gives the exercise the appearance of wave-like motion. A constant process of undulation and fluctuation.

Through practice of the solo form you learn how to precede each move in any direction with its opposite. This is important because through such practice you will learn how to use your opponent's force against him when you learn the two-person and fighting exercises. You will also learn how to defeat the opponent mentally as well as physically because in practical terms this means that a strike low will be followed by an attack high and so on. In this way the opponent will not be able to get used to pain in any one area for there will always be a point of pain somewhere else.

What this advice also reminds you of is the importance of "swing and return", whereby at the end of every movement there is a change of direction, almost like a change of gear before you move to the next posture. Thus the momentum gathered up from one movement is halted and the resulting potential energy is then used in the next move.

The mind is the commander, the qi the flag, and the waist the banner.

What this passage points to is the importance of the external being controlled by the internal. The body must be controlled by the mind and not vice-versa. The imagery here is of a military chain of command and once again it points to the fact that the qi is controlled by the mind; where you think, the qi goes. That the qi then gives commands to the waist emphasises how much you must try to use the smallest amount of muscular effort in all of your movements.

What is left unstated but is implied is that the waist in turn controls the limbs. In order to clarify this, imagine that the body is composed of a series of different-sized, interlocking cogs. The waist is the largest of these and any movements it makes are carried out through each of the other cogs : the shoulder and hip joints; the knee and elbow joints; and the ankle and wrist joints. None of these cogs, however, may be moved independently of the large cog of the waist - this in turn is motivated by the qi and therefore ultimately by the mind.

This process may best be illustrated by an examination of the opening leg and arm movements of the form. As you stand in a position of loose attention your mind runs through the mental checklist ensuring that the body is prepared to conform to the tai chi principles. Then the mind sinks the qi to the dantian (the waist region) and the movement begins, with each leg movement originating in the waist area. The arm movements are then conducted in the same manner. All the time you ensure that the whole process is slow and gradual enough that each movement segment is led by the mind; that is it is imagined fractionally before it is actually carried out.

What we are striving for here is not the total absence of muscle-power for that would be impossible, but rather making the most efficient use of the smallest amount possible. This allows tremendously powerful explosions of movement should they be necessary, for muscular reactions are fastest and most powerful when employed from a relaxed state. By performing the movements slowly and relying on the mind to direct each movement you are enabled to eliminate all unnecessary tension that would otherwise impede the swift use of total body strength.

Differentiate the substantial and insubstantial.

This is a very important maxim for the tai chi student and one that may be applied in a number of different ways. The most obvious way is related to the concept of double-weightedness. Throughout the form the majority of the weight is placed on one leg at a time. This enables you to move freely and easily. The leg with the weight on it is substantial while the other is insubstantial.

Differentiation of substantial and insubstantial, however, may also be applied to other parts of the body. This is why it is important that you know some of the possible applications for each move. Take for example the move Diagonal Flying, the lower hand is substantial, while the raised hand is insubstantial. That is, your attention is focussed on the lower hand because it is grasping and pulling down an opponent while the other hand is released to fly up and strike them.

If this differentiation is not made then your movements will be clumsy and slow and you will not be able to make use of the principle of constant change which lies at the root of the tai chi philosophy.

Use four ounces to deflect a thousand pounds

While this statement relates directly to the two-person training exercises of tai chi it is also useful when approaching form practice. This reminds you that every movement should be carried out with lightness and sensitivity.

Stand like a balance and rotate like a wheel

This advice may be directly related to the passage above as it highlights the sensitive feeling you should have while practising. It also relates to the importance of establishing a clear discrimination between the substantial and the insubstantial.

Also contained within this sentence are two important elements of form practice. One is the ability to maintain central equilibrium, the essential stability which is the foundation of each posture. The other is the constant circular movement of the form.

The spirit is relaxed and the body is calm

Once again the theme of the internal controlling the external is expressed. By relaxing the spirit the body becomes calm and thus you are able to attain the relaxation and control which are the foundation of the art.

What is meant by spirit here is best described as your thinking process, whether logical or emotional. So it might be paraphrased as calming the mind and quieting the body.

In practical terms relaxing the spirit can be achieved through the simple expedient of "sinking the qi to the dantian", or focussing the mind on one point.

Seek the straight in the curve, store and release

We are accustomed to thinking of the tai chi form in terms of curves and circles but this passage advises us to go beyond, looking for the straight line in the circle.

In fact you have already practised the straight lines of tai chi in your basic form practice when every move is broken down into its constituent parts and practised "by numbers".

The danger arises when you become too concerned with flowing, circular movements and lose the straight lines which provide the stability essential to sound posture.

The second half of this sentence is closely connected with the Cheng Man Ching principle of "swing and return", for the form consists of a constant process of storing up energy in one movement and then releasing it into the next.

Using this advice you can examine the whole of the form as you practice, finding not only the straight lines but also the points where you gather up and then release power.

Such careful analysis of the form will enable you to better understand the use of force when you come on to practising the two-person exercises.

Store up power like drawing a bow

Once again the image of storing, gathering and drawing a bow is used. As I have stated before the form is a constant process of storing and releasing power.

The more you can consciously practise this process of storing and release, the better you will be able to make use of it when you come to practising the two person exercises.

Be still like a mountain, move like a great river

This advice has already been given but it is worth repeating for the grandeur of the imagery used can inspire the feeling you will need to make your tai chi truly rooted.

When in motion everything moves, when in stillness everything is still

This is very important to your practice of the solo form as it reminds you not only that the body works as a whole unit but also that the movement of one part of has an effect on every other part of the body.

Only by gaining the ability to differentiate between relaxation and tension can you learn how to be truly still or truly in motion.

PART FOUR

SIGNPOSTS FOR THE PATH

Having completed the tai chi form your journey has only just begun and ahead of you lie many years of practice and research. Although the Cheng Man Ching form appears simple and straight-forward, such are the wide range of demands placed on both body and mind that every time you practise is a new experience.

The range of classical advice offered in the previous section is by no means comprehensive precisely because it is, and should be **your** voyage of discovery.

Finally to wave you off on your journey and hopefully to provide some signposts, I have included advice on form practice from some of the masters who have shared their knowledge with me.

NG KIONG HIN

Tai chi form is the alphabet of the art. At first we learn single letters, then we make words, then sentences, then paragraphs and so on.

But when we become more advanced it also serves as a dictionary. The dedicated student of tai chi should constantly refer back to the form to check things that they are learning. This is because when you are taught the san shou or indeed the weapons it is presumed that you have internalised the principles of the art and therefore any movement should contain tai chi. So it is that our stances are more free in the san shou and there is a danger, if you are not careful, of losing tai chi. That is when you refer to your solo form. The form keeps you on the right track.

I am not one of those teachers who thinks that the actual physical movements of the form are to be used, as they stand, for self-defence. What we can be sure of is that all the principles needed for effective self-defence are embodied in these movements. For example the turning of the waist, sinking of the hips, the ability to root et cetera.

The form develops "root". If the form is your alphabet, then "rooting" could be compared to learning to hold the pen. It is at the very foundation of our art.

What do I mean by root? I mean the ability to sink our weight into the ground in such a way that if we were to receive an incoming force we could direct it into the ground and then use it back against the opponent.

Only by learning how to relax the whole body through practising the form can we feel the connections in the body that allow force to be directed into one or other of the feet. These connections are the joints, which we try to open when we practise. It is the elasticity of the sinews which provide the force for our counter. This is tai chi's principle of "borrowing" the opponent's strength.

How then will you know that your root is being developed? At first you will know if this is working by the messages your body is giving you. If you feel discomfort in the legs then it is starting to work. The lower down the aching is, the better. You'll know when you're really feeling it when it is the bottom of your feet and your ankles that are aching.

Of course this feeling is, at this stage, subjective, to put your ability to the test you must work with a partner. This may be done first of all by having your partner push you as you run through the form.

Another important aspect of form practice is that it helps us to develop softness. To practise softness, to strive to develop relaxation is a return to our roots as human beings. Babies and small children are soft and natural. We must try to regain this state so that we can obey the principle of out of the greatest softness comes the greatest hardness. It is not easy for us human beings to be soft but it is easy to be hard. Tai chi is an internal martial art, that is it relies on sensitivity and the development of intelligent strength, not just brute force and ignorance. Unless we can be soft we cannot be sensitive; without sensitivity we cannot detect the opponent's weakness and so make intelligent use of our strength.

When we practise the form we move slowly so that we can get every movement just right and also so that we can feel the air around us. Our body becomes sensitive to everything around us.

So it is that the form provides the foundation by developing both root and softness.

TAN CHING NGEE

The first concern of the tai chi student when practising the form must be the improvement of health. At first you must relax the mind. This alone will result in the elimination of many potential ills. Western medicine now recognises the mental cause of many diseases.

Physically the constant movement from one leg to another, with the insistence on differentiation of the substantial and insubstantial, improves the circulation.

When practising the form you must take great care that you make the distinction between being relaxed and limp. Your movements must contain an alert intent. At the same time you must sink the qi to the dantian and strengthen your legs.

However far you progress with your study of tai chi you will always come back to the form so it is important that each time you practise you do so with great care and precision. Cheng Laoshi constantly stressed the importance of relaxation and was fond of telling how Yang Cheng Fu would repeat the word relax over and over again.

Tai chi is an art based on definite principles and these are all there to be discovered and explored in the form. As a teacher I can only point the way, it is up to the student to follow those signs and carry on further down the road.

If you pay attention to relaxation and the use of the waist then you will be on the right track. In addition you must always bear in mind the tai chi symbol and examine all aspects of the art in the light of this. For example each part of the body has a yin aspect and a yang aspect as does every movement and it is up to the individual student to research this through his own practice.

Tai chi chuan reflects the philosophy of constant change,

thus the art is not fixed. It will always evolve. Every student discovers this through their form practice for as one part relaxes another part will be discovered to be tense and so the process of relaxation will start all over again. This is what the art is all about and the only answers lie in training and research.

LAU KIM HONG

In Cheng Man Ching style tai chi chuan the unique characteristic and major emphasis is on "song". Master Cheng used all his experience to encapsulate all the skill of tai chi in one concept- "song". By so doing he has saved us all from following the wrong road. Unfortunately there have been too many books on the art written by people who are intent on feeding their families and so they write all sorts of nonsense about things of which they have no personal experience. Cheng Man Ching was not like that, his books contain his own experience. Anything that he wrote about he had personally experienced.

Over the years that I have been studying tai chi I have brought hundreds of books but they are full of "blind alleys". Some books say that your attitude of mind when doing the form should be as if you were fighting someone. This is a "blind alley". Someone has taken the theories of Shaolin boxing and applied them to tai chi. But in tai chi our first consideration must be "song". You don't relax by thinking you are about to be attacked, instead you will get tense, excited and nervous.

When we practise the form the movements are very extended and open, this is to aid relaxation and to promote good health. That doesn't mean we actually fight with our arms open wide.

As to the precise amount of time that you should spend in practice each day, that very much depends on the amount of time available to you. Allow your practice to proceed naturally, just a few minutes a day will do to begin with. When you first start training your physical limitations will determine how long you can practise. Your knees and ankles will ache, your legs will tremble and so on. But once you've acquired some strength then you will practise the form with larger steps to further train your legs so that once again your physical limitations will determine the duration of your practice and so the cycle continues.

In order to ascertain whether your form is correct you must check the advice given in the "classics". You have to constantly check to determine whether you are following the tai chi principles. The most basic of these are pieces of advice like keep the head erect, hollow the chest and round the shoulders. All of these, however, are natural. Of course it's better if you have a teacher who can give you advice and stop you wandering up too many "blind alleys".

Your most important motive for training the form should be to train "song". If you are not "song" and "chen" (sunk) then you will be forced to rely on brute strength when it comes to pushing hands and fighting applications. One important distinction that must be made is between "song" and "ruan" (the softness of cooked spaghetti). If you are "song" but not "chen", then in my opinion you are "ruan", and this is not a quality that is part of tai chi chuan. If you are "song" and "chen" then you will have acquired central equilibrium which is one of the major aims of form practice.

KOH AH TEE

The most important purpose of form training is to relax the sinews; this must be first and foremost. From relaxation of the sinews comes relaxation of the muscles and so the whole body.

Its other purposes are to connect mind, heart, qi and body. Use the mind to control the heart; the heart controls the qi and the qi moves the body. Tai chi chuan is not a question of moving the hand or foot on their own, instead it is the qi that is the motivating force, the qi moves the limbs.

In addition in tai chi we strive to allow the lower body to control the upper body. That is the power is derived from the yong quan. "The power is rooted in the feet, directed by the legs, controlled by the waist and expressed through the arms", as it says in the "classics .

If you look at the film evidence of Grandmaster Cheng's career you can see quite clearly that the older he got the more relaxed he became. This is inevitable because as I have said before tai chi turns things on their head, it does not rely on natural strength, so that as the grandmaster got older all he had to rely on was qi.

Tai Chi is different from external martial arts which rely on brute strength. When you get old and there is no strength left then you have to rely on a different kind of gong fu. When he got older, as you could see in his pushing hands, there was no longer any preparation, when people touched him they flew away!

The form can be seen as a compendium of the strategy and tactics of the art. If we look at two specific movements, Jing Bu Ban Lan Chui and Lou Xi Ao Bu we can see how this works.

In the first when punching we do so to the centre of the body, the soft parts. In the second we use the open hand to the face or chest, both hard parts. We are using Yin against Yang and Yang against Yin. But also if we look at the body mechanics and the laws of physics involved we can see that to punch high is unnatural in the sense that it requires tension in the shoulders and the upper body; a high open-hand strike, on the other hand is both relaxed and natural. This is the reason for the difference and this same reasoning in terms of application may be applied to every movement in the form.

When I am teaching I explain every movement in terms of application, but I don't think that it is important to give students opportunities to practise these moves. The reason for this is that fighting is not a question of my opponent uses this method so I use that method. If it is not natural it is not tai chi. You relax and wait for the opponent. He moves first but you arrive first. When the students have an understanding of the applications and practise them in the form, they allow them to become internalised so that they become natural reactions not trained responses, reacting to an external stimuli.

Once they become internalised and are combined with relaxation you will have the ability to calmly wait and respond. Standing with a puffed-up chest and wide-staring eyes is not tai chi, that is a case of putting on a bold exterior while what we really want is a strong interior.

This is my own belief but it should not be a case of me telling you so that you **must** believe it. No, you should think for yourself, put these ideas to the test. These are the result of my years of experience but I cannot make anyone believe them, they have to be experienced.

Grandmaster Cheng himself wrote to the effect that when you know the essence of tai chi, you will be able to use it. When the time is right understanding comes like a flash of enlightenment.

But let me tell you the best thing about tai chi is that it curbs your temper, calm you down. You are less-inclined to get in a fight because someone says you have no skill. If you find that you still have a tendency to lose your temper then your gong fu hasn't yet got to the highest level. If there is going to be a fight both people have to want it, if you apologise or step back there is no fight!

Tai chi is a form of self-cultivation.